*my*fibromyalgia

one man's experience of living with chronic illness

Andrew Hinkinson

Published by Andrew Hinkinson 2018

www.andrewhinkinson.com
Cover design by the author.

ISBN-13: 978-1-9829953-1-7

Other books by the same author

Non-fiction
Chickens As Pets - Your Definitive Guide to
Keeping Pet Chickens

Fiction
Woof!

About the author

Andrew Hinkinson has a copywriting and editing career spanning two decades. He has a Bachelor's degree in English and Theatre from Goldsmiths College, University of London and an MA in Creative Writing from Manchester Metropolitan University. He lives in the Yorkshire Dales, England.

myfibromyalgia is Andrew's second non-fiction title and his third book. Andrew has fibromyalgia, keeps pet chickens and cats, loves *Doctor Who* and comics, and maintains an author presence online with Tumblr, Twitter, Facebook and his personal website. Start connecting with him via andrewhinkinson.com.

This book is dedicated to all the fibro warriors around the world.

Acknowledgements

I'd like to take the opportunity to thank you for buying this book and thank my fellow FMS warriors who generously shared their own stories and gave me permission to quote them - Debbie, Sharon, Michael, Katy, Kelly and Luke. My gratitude extends as well to those in the medical profession who have treated me, talked with me, helped me build my own post-diagnosis future and informed my understanding of fibromyalgia.

Without my mother and late father always being there for me, I don't think I would have had the courage and determination to forge a path in life for myself that was fundamentally my own choice, to pursue a career in manifesting words on paper and screen. I always wanted to be a writer. When I wasn't wanting to be an astronaut or cartoonist. But hey.

Thanks to my friend Killian Broadley for helping me on occasions with the day to day stuff that can be impossible for fibro sufferers to do alone. Thank you also to my kind friend, Soo Feather, for taking on the role of 'foster mum' to my pet chickens and turkeys to help me out when I recognised I was trying to do everything but couldn't.

Contents

Introduction

I'm Andrew. I'm a writer. I'm not a doctor or a nurse or any other medical professional. I have fibromyalgia (FMS - the S stands for 'syndrome'). At time of writing this, I've had my diagnosis of FMS for five years.

When the seed of this book took root inside my head, I'd had a terrible night of trying and failing to get much sleep, thanks to chronic pain in my hands, arms and legs waking me up almost hourly. This wasn't unusual; it was, and remains, common for me to suffer disturbed sleep and insomnia. I gave up on the hope of getting anything like half-decent sleep around 4.30am. I knew I would doze during the day, fitfully, maybe a couple of times, ten or twenty minutes here and there. Dozing is no substitute for good quality sleep but when you're in pain you'll take what you can get. It's one thing for doctors to advise against snatching forty winks in the day if you want to sleep at night but they assume that, by not catnapping, you'll sleep when your proper bedtime comes round. And that's not a given.

So anyway, there I was, lying in bed, thinking. What else was I supposed to do when I was hurting and wide awake? My FMS symptoms had been really, really bad for some time. They come, for all sufferers, in peaks and troughs lasting days, weeks or even months before dipping or rising again. A few days earlier I'd made the discovery that I couldn't open an envelope that morning, a new frustration. I'd long before then learned that unscrewing a bottle was an impossibility - but a frickin' envelope? Seriously? My hands were often like paddles before noon, useful if I was ever to find myself without an oar in a boat on a lake, I guess, but sod all use in any other context. This book will detail the many (oh so many, way too many) FMS symptoms and their variability as you read on; let's focus for now on why I decided to write about this strange disability in the first place.

After abandoning all hope of sleep on the aforementioned night, I searched online for information on FMS, not for the first time. Just to see if there were any new ideas on how to treat it. Progress in confirming causes, let alone any prospect of a cure, is slow. Medical researchers need controls, safeguards against bias, standardised laboratory conditions and peer reviews of work. You know, things that take us beyond the 'suck it and see' philosophy or its close relative, 'I did this and got better, so the reason must be the thing I did' - which, examined logically, would mean if you get better from a cold after a crow shits on your car windscreen, you'll be begging those big, magnificent birds to crap on your vehicle come the next flu season. I frequently encounter people who join the dots and see causality where there is none. It's a human thing, hardwired into us back when we lived in trees.

With FMS there's a heck of a lot of tosh, some of it potentially harmful, in the form of advice available to read online, on webpages and in forums. Things that can't be proven scientifically but sound great to anyone, not least those of us desperate to find something, anything, to stop the pain. I want to have confidence in my treatments, though. I want medical professionals with years of training to have a cure for me. I don't want to hand over responsibility for changing my life to someone with a marketing plan to earn themselves a fortune, and unverifiable testimonies. There are hundreds of thousands of people the world over who suffer terrible pain and are insulted at best, misled at worst, by fake news and bogus health websites, self-styled wellness gurus and the (thankfully diminishing number of) doubters, including some doctors, who rank FMS alongside fairies, the Loch Ness Monster and UFOs. Fibromyalgia is probably second to cancer for attracting all sorts of kookiness online and strange rumblings from within the medical profession. I wanted to write a book that told the truth, from the perspective of a patient rather than a doctor. A book about what it's like to live with FMS.

There are no miracle cures on offer here. I'm not going to try to sell you a course. No, no, no. That's not what this is about at all. What you're going to read as you make your way through this book is an honest and frank account with opinions and ideas expressed without any suggestion that I've got the answers or even want to be the guy people turn to thinking I'll tell them what to do. I don't, and I won't. This book doesn't touch upon all of the theories, all of the possible drugs and treatments, all of the ideas in all of the world about and pertaining to FMS. It couldn't, not without being a massive multi-volume collection of books packed with incredible detail only medical practitioners could fully grasp. It's a personal account. My fibromyalgia. No one else's. My aim isn't to befuddle you with jargon. I'm going to keep everything as simple as possible, explaining as I go. I throw in some humour every now and then, because this isn't a bland textbook that has to be devoid of personality but the living, breathing testimony of a real FMS sufferer. I want you to find this reading experience as entertaining as it is informative. If I haven't touched upon something, it's because it hasn't touched me, at least not yet.

This book gives people who don't have FMS, but perhaps know others who do, insight into what it is like to live with it. It sends a message of 'you're not alone' to the many FMS sufferers who do feel alone. Some of them might think they're losing their minds. It's easy to think like that, when you've got nobody to compare to, and no idea what the strange symptoms you're manifesting are all about, what they signify. A lot of FMS sufferers are undiagnosed and/or finding it hard to get doctors, family and friends to take their condition seriously. You. Are. Not. Alone.

I swear, just a little, in these pages from time to time. Be advised. This is real. This is me. Like I've already told you, this is no dry manual. It's my lived, truthful experience and I'm a bloke who swears, especially when I'm in great pain or frustrated and angry at this horrible disability that seemed to come at me from nowhere. If you're the kind of person who can say "Golly gumdrops!" after dropping a huge weight on your toe, I'm pleased for you but I'm not that kind of guy. If (very light) swearing offends you, then (a) you've got every right to stop reading, and (b) if you have FMS and your biggest concern is other people using swear words in books, I'm really impressed. I'm not sure why I'm impressed, but I am. I guess my point is: people are inclined to cuss when things go bad. FMS is one of the very bad things, no doubt about that, and so it makes me sweary.

The pain is real and constant. I eat well, I exercise when I can, I fight this thing called fibromyalgia every day. Even so, it's driven a wrecking ball through my hopes, my dreams, my ambitions - and still I keep on hoping, dreaming, aiming for the sky. I'm stubborn that way.

When disabilities of any kind are discussed, what you're really talking about are people: flesh and blood, breathing, thinking, feeling people. We are all different. We share symptoms but our experiences in life, beliefs and lifestyles are unique to each of us.

Welcome to *my*fibromyalgia.

In the beginning

I'd love to start at the beginning because Julie Andrews told me in 'The Sound of Music', every Christmas on TV since I was a small child to the present day, that it's a very good place to start. She was right, was Julie.

The thing is, I don't know exactly where - or when - my fibromyalgia story starts, not really. When I finally got a diagnosis, I was surprised by a question put to me by my consultant (I'll refer to him as Dr G).

"What other symptoms have you had, even going back as long ago as ten years or more? Strange things."

Well, I thought. This whole situation with my health is strange, but okay…

It turned out, some of the health issues I'd lived with for years had been symptoms of the illness. For at least a decade I'd suffered occasionally from what I referred to as 'closing doors' in my oesophagus. I'd be eating something and there'd be this feeling of doors swishing shut, from side to side, just like in 'Star Trek'. One by one, each of these imagined doors would close, starting at the top of my throat and going all the way down to my stomach. I could even count them, six or seven doors, the number wasn't entirely, perfectly fixed from one attack to the next.

I knew I wasn't imagining these feelings of interior shutdown. It was as if my oesophagus was flattening like a punctured tyre. When it first happened, I can't recall exactly when, I went into a panic. I dropped my knife and fork and began to do an impression of a goldfish out of water. I wasn't really thinking, not in that moment. If there was anything like a thought, it was: I'm suffocating.

After several minutes of not dying, my throat opened for business again. I didn't much feel like eating or drinking for a while afterwards, though.

It was a few months before I was hit by the same weird symptom again. The second time I knew I wasn't going to die and didn't need an ambulance or any drama around me. I just put my knife and fork down, leaned back away from the table, and waited calmly for it to stop. That last part is easy to write down, not so easy to achieve. But I did it. And, surely enough, after a few minutes, the mysterious grip on my oesophagus relaxed. This time, I did start eating and drinking again - slowly, thoughtfully, chewing that little bit more before swallowing, thinking it might help. It certainly didn't make things any worse.

My partner at the time asked if it was because I'd been bolting my food but no. It wasn't, because I didn't bolt my food, not ever. When I eventually told my GP about the symptom - it was happening on an irregular basis, sometimes weeks apart but more often months - she wrote me a prescription for an inhaler and said I had asthma.

Like hell, I thought. I don't have asthma. Still, I dutifully tried using the inhaler and it did absolutely diddly-squat to alleviate the frequency and intensity of the attacks. Besides, I couldn't use it when one of them was upon me, all internal doors swishing closed. It was all I could do, in that situation, to keep my head from going into full-on "WE'RE ALL GOING TO DIE! RUN FOR THE HILLS!" mode. The last thing I could think of was reaching for the inhaler. Heck, thinking wasn't really happening at all.

"That," said Dr G, leaning back in his chair and scrutinising me like a bug under a microscope, "is a symptom of fibromyalgia. Patients with fibromyalgia often report it."

A light-bulb moment! All of a sudden, some small part of the weirdness that was me made a little more sense than it had before I turned up that day for my hospital appointment.

I guess my oesophagus acting so strangely, that might have been the starting gun fired, the opening salvo for FMS. The chronic pain from head to toe, the sleep disturbance, the chronic fatigue, the brain fog (confused thoughts, inability to keep track of conversations)… All of those started to hit me several years after my inside gut doors had begun to mess with my meal times. They didn't all come at once, I remember that much. The pain and stiffness, they were the last symptoms to materialise. They did so immediately after a short but intense flu. One theory about FMS involves flu viruses getting into the spine but I'm not going to say that happened to me. I don't know and I don't think I ever will know exactly why I developed fibromyalgia. We know some possible causes but we know it isn't likely FMS results from just one thing – and we don't know why some people are unaffected by things that in others result in this painful, mysterious malady. Maybe science will one day come up with a definitive answer and an effective, lasting treatment. I really hope so. That day is a long way off, though, and we all have to do what we can in the meantime.

Symptoms

In these days of Google being the go-to for everything under the sun, from facts to half-baked opinions to outright fake news, it's easy to get information about anything that ails you. Whether that information is true or false, that's something to ponder, and to date Google hasn't had the audacity to set itself up as an arbiter of truth. Give it time, though.

No, Google is more like a guide who can take you on a tour of the city, pointing at this building or that, but isn't actually able to tell you anything about what you're seeing. For that, you have to go inside and find out for yourself, or ask the dodgy-looking guy on the street corner to tell his story for the price of a pint.

There's no guarantee information you come across online is true. The internet encourages us to hop from site to site, page to page, by way of hyperlinks, forging connections in our minds that may or may not lead us down strange and dangerous paths.

If you're a particular kind of person, you might end up convincing yourself that you've got cancer of the genitals, a rare tropical disease that eats the brain, and fibromyalgia. All from spending fifteen minutes using a search engine. Even if you aren't a hypochondriac or easily scared, the symptoms of an illness are often duplicated with countless other illnesses - a cough, for example, or a rash. We need doctors to pin down what's wrong with us. Even doctors need other doctors when they're sick, because self-diagnosis is a bad idea even for the medically qualified.

Even though it's a condition about which little is known or agreed upon, FMS has a lot of pages devoted to it online. These are made public by legitimate, proven publishers of generally reliable information - such as the UK's National Health Service - and then there's the material put out by altogether more colourful, rich individuals running 'alternative' health empires and posting YouTube videos about how much they want to heal the world while driving massive cars their followers and advertisers pay for.

It's not my aim to discourage the use of herbal remedies, acupuncture and other so-called non-mainstream treatments. Many of them do actually work, somehow, whether the effect is that of a placebo - mind over matter - or down to some as yet unknown mechanism. I would, though, urge you to exercise caution. Deploy your critical faculties to the full when assessing all the claims put out there, for both causes of FMS and 'cures' for it. Before you know it, you can spend a lot of your hard-earned money, getting nowhere but poorer. You might end up eating shedloads of spinach because Dr Miracle told you it cures every ailment known to humanity. Spinach is good for you, sure, in general nutritional terms. I love the stuff but I've yet to get muscles like Popeye. Eating a lot of it isn't going to damage you, assuming you're not allergic to it. Hokey ideas other than eating more of a certain vegetable can, however, be potentially harmful and even life-limiting. Taking someone on trust when they say spinach can cure FMS or cancer can also be psychologically damaging when, inevitably, it doesn't do what you were promised it would. In the case of quack cancer treatments, they can result in death.

I'm writing about FMS without the flim-flam of the snake oil seller. You won't get the impossible-to-understand detail of the specialist, either, who forgets his or her audience in a consulting room doesn't have a medical degree. At its simplest, FMS is a long-term, chronic illness that involves pain being felt throughout the body. Chronic is a word people associate with a high level of intensity ("It's chronic today!" meaning "It's hurting me real bad, so I've got a short temper and will end you if you annoy me!") but it actually means something that is persistent (doesn't go away). If you play the word association game with a FMS sufferer and say 'fibro' to them, their response is most likely to be 'pain'. That's what springs to our minds, first and foremost.

In no particular order, because all the symptoms are equally horrible and very difficult to live with, the symptoms of FMS are as follows:

Pain. Pain is the ultimate swear-generator. It is the evil git, the monster, the muthafafaowowow. It assaults us from head to toe, stabbing, burning its way across our skin and through our nervous system, our muscles, the backs of our eyes. We have headaches, sickness, feel inflamed, our joints ache, there are feelings like hot needles being shoved down our fingertips, into our wrists, our knees, our ankles. We get chest pain, bowel pain, stomach pain, ball pain, ovary pain... Some days are better than others. Some are the worst they could be. You can't communicate to anyone else how bad your pain is, either. It's subjective - unknowable from one person to another. Even with doctors, we can only give them an idea of how bad it is for us. They can't truly know.

Feeling knackered all the time. The official word to describe this is 'fatigue' and you'll often hear 'chronic fatigue' mentioned in relation to FMS. I've yet to meet anyone with fibro who doesn't have to deal with fatigue just as much as pain.

Not getting a decent night's sleep. This isn't so much insomnia, because you can get to sleep, usually, eventually, sort of. Just not when you want to. It's constantly interrupted sleep, that's the issue, and it's all thanks to the pain kicking you awake at intervals throughout the night. I get shooting pains in my hands, arms and legs that guarantee I wake up every two hours or so. This means deep sleep is harder to come by, which is a bad thing with a cumulative effect of screwing you over good and proper. Sure, if you aren't at work on any given day or unable to work at all, you can nap during the day but it isn't like the proper sleep you're supposed to be getting. That's why we call it a nap: sleep lite, rather than sleep+.

Drugs are often prescribed to ease us into sleep and keep us there, and they work to stop us waking in response to the stabbing and searing pains that assault us. Amitriptyline is one I've got experience of using, an antidepressant no longer generally prescribed for that purpose but for its tranquillising effect. Amitriptyline does work: you will get a full night of sleep. The problem I found, and which everyone finds, with this drug is that you wake the next day feeling like someone shoved cotton wool up your bum in the night and stuffed it all the way up your digestive system, into your mouth and brain. And that leads me onto the next symptom,

Brain fog or 'fibro fog' or "I'm totally messed up in the head today". The polite description of this phenomenon associated with FMS is something along the lines of 'memory and concentration problems' but, really, as with so many medical textbook phrasings, that is lovely and succinct and does nothing to actually relay what it's like to experience. The drugs, like the aforementioned amitriptyline, can make this extreme wooly-headedness worse but they don't cause it. It's a symptom of the illness.

It doesn't matter how old you are, if you have FMS you'll find yourself having 'senior moments' every day: you forget your umbrella and realise when you're five minutes into being outside the house in the pouring rain, when you finally notice you're getting wet; you listen intently to a friend detailing how their date went, then realise you didn't actually listen at all, and went somewhere else in your head that you don't remember anything about, somewhere around their third sentence, you think but you can't be sure... You will annoy friends and family if you have FMS, for various reasons but most certainly when they think you aren't paying attention to them. Because what everyone has to say to you is always important, after all. Even if it's only asking you to get some milk.

Feeling as stiff as a corpse laid out in the funeral home. I call my morning self the Tin Man, because I wake and it takes me anywhere from half an hour to three hours to stop walking around like I'm rusty and in need of a full-body oil change and joint lubrication. Pills of any kind won't hurry this process of daily resurrection along. Believe me, I take my Omega-3 oil (extracted from algae, not fish, because I don't eat fish or meat), calcium, vitamin D and all the rest of the supplements said to help us move with less pain. Most days I do, eventually, come round.

On days when the FMS is going to beat my body good and proper to show me it's in charge, the struggle never goes away and it's a battle to get out of bed and do much of anything. Not moving doesn't make the pain go away, though. It's better to grit your teeth, swear a lot and fight to move around and get a little bit done even if your list of to-dos for the day goes out the window. It's just, you know, some days are bad days emotionally because of this rotten illness and you do, inevitably, give up on those days. Don't beat yourself up if that happens. You're only human. Tomorrow is a new day and the sooner it comes, the better.

Headaches. Yeah, there's no need to wax lyrical about these. They are what they are. They vary in intensity. Some FMS sufferers get migraines all the time. It's the one aspect I've struck lucky on, in that I get migraines 'only' a few times a month. Whoopee for me. I'm so blessed. Some poor souls get them every day. It could be that our posture makes these happen, or makes them worse, because we tend to hold ourselves in less than optimal positions when we're dealing with intense pain in this or that limb, or all our limbs. I'm including the neck, which isn't a limb but does feel the hurt just the same as elbows, knees and every other damn place that has bones in it. Which is all of you.

Poops as inconsistent as politicians' statements from one day to the next. Irritable Bowel Syndrome (IBS) is the label we apply to the stomach pain, bloating, and strange goings-on in Toilet Land. You can eat a diet any doctor would award you five gold stars for - high fibre, unprocessed foods, plenty of vegetables and fruit, enough water to fill a tank - and still find yourself either suffering from diarrhoea or constipation, or both alternately, and rarely enjoy the comfort of the middle, altogether firmer, zone.

As part of their ongoing investigations into something they're generally clueless about, our doctors send us for colonoscopies and gastroscopies. These are, to be fair, necessary in order to rule out cancers and generally benign but obstructive growths called polyps. The procedures involve tortures you thought were put an end to when the Inquisition was forced to put out the fires, stop the hangings and retire those beautifully crafted instruments of torture now displayed in museums. Doctors will play around with your diet, advocating no fibre, more fibre, gluten-free, dairy-free. Some of their advice when taken will help. Some of it won't.

The simple fact is, FMS is shit and messes with your shit, big time. You learn to buy soft, good quality toilet paper in quantity, never allow yourself to run out of it and always have good reading material close by in the bathroom. As for the pain involved, which can be immense, there are bowel analgesics you can be prescribed, which mask the problem and allow you to walk around like a person rather than crawl like Gollum in Lord of the Rings. Oh, and you can guarantee a flat stomach all day until you're just about to go out on that hot date, or anywhere you want to look your best, when your tummy will inflate to give the impression you're five months pregnant. Even if you're a man.

My own situation with IBS is complicated by a condition called diverticulosis or diverticular disease, where the lower bowel is pockmarked inside, with pouches, like deep craters on the moon. This can result in diverticulitis, which is when one or more of those pouches get infected. In my case, this was likely caused by a drug I was wrongly prescribed as a treatment for FMS - a steroid called Prednisone (also known as Prednisolone), long-term use of which (I was left on it for four years, unchecked) can damage the bowel lining. Yeah, I know. There's nothing you can say I haven't wanted to scream about this.

Causes

Many a doctor has, at one time or another, come up with theories as to what causes fibromyalgia. The problem with theories tends to be that some patients can nod and recognise they've been through certain illnesses and experiences thought to lead to the onset of FMS, while others won't connect at all to whatever cause is being put forward. There isn't, as yet, one overarching theory to encompass the many possible causes. By that, I mean there may be a commonality among FMS sufferers as yet unidentified but what's certain is that not everyone who suffers, say, a traumatic accident or assault goes on to develop the syndrome. One possible cause is the death of a loved one. Everyone goes through that sooner or later, so why do only some people develop FMS in response to it? FMS does appear to be triggered or made worse, for many people, by physically and/or emotionally stressful events in their lives. Me, I've no doubt at all getting stressed makes my FMS symptoms worse. What isn't known is what makes some people develop FMS in response to various stressors while others don't.

You'll hear talk of triggers in discussions around FMS. These are the emotional and physical events in your life thought to be partly responsible for bringing on the symptoms of FMS or, if you already have it, making it worse. It's important to recognise that triggers alone can't be said to be wholly responsible, because many of them are experienced by lots of people who don't get ill as a consequence. There's evidently something else going on inside FMS sufferers as well. People can and do theorise until the cows come home as to what the magic ingredient might be that makes us more likely to develop FMS, from the food we eat to the lifestyles we lead, the air we breathe and events in childhood.

The triggers for a FMS response can include:

The breakdown of a relationship. He dumped you but did he need to be a total dick about it and make you homeless at the same time, leaving you with the six cats you both signed up to care for seven years earlier? Or, she walked away with the guy who works at the corner shop and left you with a mortgage to pay all on your own, but keeping things going will be a struggle and you don't know how you're going to afford to pay for food and settle your bills. There are so many horror story variants when it comes to relationships ending. The point is, there are ways and means of ending relationships. Some can be ended fairly gently, with mutual respect and accord that it's over; others can end with recriminations, violent arguments and shockingly bad behaviour of one ex-partner towards the other. The harder the break, the more impactful it is, psychologically and, undoubtedly, physically as well. I'm absolutely convinced a traumatic break-up was responsible for FMS fully manifesting in my life, although I'd been displaying some but not all symptoms for some years before the split happened.

The death of a loved one. This can be a mother, a father, a friend, a child. It can be a pet you've loved for ten years. The loss is felt physically, in your muscles and bones, as well as in the heart and mind. You don't eat, you don't sleep, you cry a river. Yes, these are all normal components of the grieving process but, for some, grief affects them in their bodies for much longer than it does other people. You might have moved on emotionally but your body can hurt from the loss and stress for a very long time.

Accidents. They might involve spectacular pratfalls that land you in A&E or slicing through your finger when chopping vegetables, but accidents can have consequences that last way beyond the time it takes for bleeding bits to stop bleeding and broken bones to heal. There's a shock to the system – the trauma of an impact – and, while most people find themselves 'rattled' for only a short period of time, for those with FMS the feeling of being shook up and turned upside down sticks around like the last person at the party you wish would go home. Having operations can also upset the body for a long time when you have FMS. You're out for the count while things are done to you but it's as if the body and the brain somehow remember what your mind can't, and can go on to give you trouble long afterwards.

Post-traumatic stress disorder (PTSD) is a mental health problem resulting from the experience of traumatic events. PTSD is most often referenced in relation to soldiers who have experienced the horrors of war but can develop after being raped, surviving car accidents and going through any life-threatening or prolonged intimidating situations. FMS can develop alongside PTSD symptoms.

Abuse. Physical and psychological abuse can change the way the brain responds to perceived threats, pain and general everyday stress. Abused children are significantly more likely than their peers to develop FMS later in their lives.

Other illnesses and disorders. Arthritis, rheumatism and infections all increase your risk of developing FMS as do common mental health problems such as anxiety, depression and other mood disorders.

Sedentary lifestyles. Not moving enough, in other words. This might mean spending all your free time on the sofa but it can also involve a huge number of jobs in the modern world that have you sat at a desk pretty much all the time. I'm very much aware writing is one of those sedentary jobs, but whether my chosen career path led to me developing FMS, I've no idea. Not every writer ends up living with FMS, that's for sure. I was quite active and spent a lot of time outdoors prior to developing it. I have found exercise can help alleviate symptoms but only when they're not so intense and disabling as to totally block my ability to do much of anything physical. Even then, on good days, I have to take care not to do too much - and what constitutes too much will vary from one person to the next as well as from day to day. When I do too much exercise I'm flat on my back for days at a time afterwards. I often don't know I did too much until I wake the next day barely able to move.

Sex. I don't mean sex as in recreational and procreational intimacy, but rather male and female biology. Gender is a whole different story, being socially determined. The focus here is on the physical, not the abstract. FMS is said to affect seven times more women than it does men, but there are potentially vast numbers of unreported cases, with men far less likely than women to go the doctor when they really need to. There are also men and women with FMS who struggle for decades to get a diagnosis from doctors who don't believe the syndrome is real. In what ways FMS impacts upon us based on our biology as men and women is unknown, as is the role of gender in making us more or less likely to report to doctors that we have symptoms, and determining how we respond to pain.

Men and women often behave differently only because they're raised to believe they should act differently, rather than them being biologically predisposed to do things in specific ways. This is where gender comes in. Men are often raised to conceal their emotions, even to suppress them, and this extends to not going to see the doctor when they're in pain. If a man has all the symptoms of FMS but hears that it's a 'woman's thing', he might conclude he can't possibly have it. He could then embark upon a destructive daily routine of taking ever more powerful over-the-counter drugs until he messes up his stomach or liver or kidneys. He might only be diagnosed with FMS, if at all, after years of suffering while ineffectively and dangerously self-medicating.

A man might not go to the doctor because he thinks it's his job to soldier on. Who tells men this guff? It has to stop. Seriously. Let men be men and women be women, whatever that means for each individual, not what society tells them men and women are supposed to be. Okay, I'll get down from my soapbox now. I do believe, though, that the expectations put upon us from an early age can screw with us for our entire lives. I'll always be grateful to my parents for raising me not to suffer in silence, not to be afraid of crying and to freely express a full range of emotions.

Family. FMS isn't hereditary but it has been found to be more likely diagnosed if you already have a sibling or other relative with FMS. It's thought likely that there are certain genes which can make you more sensitive to pain and more likely to experience anxiety and depression, both of which make pain worse and increase susceptibility to other illnesses. These genes don't guarantee you'll get FMS.

There are a lot of estimates in orbit around FMS, with one of them being that 'nearly' one in 20 people might have fibro 'to some degree'. The picture isn't going to get any clearer any time soon, not while we still have doctors who don't believe FMS actually exists and it remains a condition shrouded in mystery. Even among those medical practitioners who entertain FMS as a possible diagnosis, they would all say that FMS can be a very hard condition to diagnose. Nobody wants to give a wrong diagnosis, after all, because that can have negative consequences for you and them, and there's no specific test. Okay, there's one. It involves 'pain points' around the body. The doctor basically stabs you with a pointy instrument in various places to see if you'll say "OW! THAT HURTS! STOP!" or, if you're a little sheepish around someone with a stethoscope, you might instead say, "Yes, that does hurt a little, Doctor." Reticence and politeness, though, don't do you any favours when a medical professional is poking you with a sharp stick. If it hurts, make it clear.

The test is imprecise to say the least and, while it gives patients the no doubt valuable experience of what life would be like if they were a pin cushion, it simply isn't seen anymore as an entirely reliable diagnostic tool to determine or discount a FMS diagnosis. At best, it can help a doctor move closer towards a definitive answer as to what's wrong with you. At worst, it can result in your FMS not being diagnosed because an outdated, unreliable test is being used as the only diagnostic tool. Which, sadly, does happen.

Numbers

Often, when talking to people, I get the impression they think fibromyalgia is something uncommon and, indeed, very unusual. That's simply not true. The American Chronic Pain Society (there's a society for everything these days) estimates three to six per cent of the global population has FMS. That may not seem a lot to you, but as I'm writing this I'm looking at the world population clock (you can check this out yourself at worldometers.info/world-population) and it's showing 7,616,432,212 people living on the planet. Of course, before I'd even finished typing that sentence, the number went up. And up, and up. What this means is between 200 million and 400 million people are living with FMS. Uncommon and unusual? Don't bet on it.

As many as 10 million of those people are living in the United States, although that country's National Pain Foundation believes around two per cent of its population has fibro, which works out to around three million to six million people. Other professional bodies in the US place the figure even higher, as high as eight million. The point is, it's an awful lot of people in one, admittedly very big, country to be suffering every day with a crippling, chronically painful condition for which medical science has yet to provide a fully effective treatment for, let alone a cure.

If we extrapolate from the available data and suppositions by American agencies, assuming similar percentages in other Western countries, this means around 800,000 people in the UK could have FMS. The UK's National Health Service itself estimates two to 4.5 per cent of the UK population. From a UK population of over 61 million, that works out as between 1.2 million and 2.8 million people.

The syndrome is most commonly diagnosed in white women and very little, if any, research has been conducted on FMS in Asians, Hispanics, Native Americans and black people. One theory put forward for this, and lower levels of diagnosis in these ethnic groups, is because, in those countries where comprehensive health care is only obtained by having adequate (and expensive) health insurance, people in these groups are often poorly served due to lower incomes and an inability to pay. FMS has, though, been found to impact upon different social classes and ethnicities in roughly the same proportion. A study in Israel compared Israeli women to Bedouin women and found 3.7 per cent of both equally were affected by the condition. In Canada, the prevalence of FMS within the general population was compared to that of the Amish community and, again, no significant difference was found.

Anywhere between 75 and 90 per cent of people living with FMS are female, although, as I wrote in the previous chapter, the number of men with the syndrome is likely to be underreported but not so much as to invalidate the generally correct perception of FMS as being much more common among women. The false sense, though, that it is a disorder afflicting only women and not men, is very likely why, given the rampant sexism women have had to deal with since time immemorial, FMS was dismissed and even ridiculed as make-believe for a very long time by predominantly male doctors. Female doctors weren't even sanctioned to practice for the longest time - women weren't allowed to train in medical schools - and women were involved in the medical profession as nurses on hand to assist male doctors.

We really don't have to delve that far into the past to find women with real health problems dismissed as being hysterical. Even the word, hysteria, originates from the Greek word for 'uterus'. Historically, hysteria was the word applied to women displaying a variety of symptoms that included being short of breath, fainting, unable to sleep, nervous, and irritable. Those can be symptoms of many absolutely genuine illnesses, including FMS. A woman could even be labelled hysterical if she exhibited enthusiastic sexual desire.

Many of us have this idea that doctors always know what they're talking about and, to be clear, they often, indeed usually, do. A doctor is only ever as good, though, as current medical knowledge allows them to be, and social prejudices shift and change over time. If they own those social prejudices themselves, and propagate them, or at the very least allow the fact-free bigotries of the day to inform their decision-making processes, then they aren't being quite as scientific and logical in their approaches to patient care as we would hope for them to be. We don't need to go a long way back in time to find an example of a time when medical practitioners allowed bigotry to inform their actions. Gay and bisexual men in the 1980s would often visit their doctor for any condition at all and find themselves being asked to take the HIV test, unnecessarily, based on the false assumption they would likely be HIV+ because of their sexuality. The most appalling treatment of gay and bisexual men who were HIV+ in that decade - while in hospitals, even when dying - is well-documented.

Setting aside the potential fallibility and flaws of doctors as human beings (and we can't blame them for being imperfect, because we all are), there remains in the 21st Century a great deal of what we laymen and women might call 'stuff' that medical professionals just don't know anything about. I once interviewed a brain surgeon, who told me that we know less than ten per cent of what the brain does, how it works. It doesn't mean they're winging it when they perform major brain surgery, but it does mean there's an awful lot more to learn about the second-largest organ in the human body (the top slot being occupied by the skin). FMS is a great mystery to medical minds, and there is research being undertaken all the time now to find out what it is exactly, and how to treat it.

There is no doubt whatsoever that the historical approach to FMS, certainly up to the tail end of the 20th Century, is tied up with how women have been viewed by society and the medical profession. And while more men are being diagnosed with the syndrome, it isn't this fact which has resulted in it being taken more seriously, it's a combination of women's rights being advanced and, most of all, by those with symptoms regardless of their sex not going away, not getting better and, if anything, increasing in numbers. As this chapter has already shown, the numbers afflicted are significant. They are huge.

FMS symptoms generally start between the ages of 20 and 55, although juvenile instances of the development of the syndrome are increasingly being identified and paid attention to, although children can't choose to participate in research studies, not until they reach adulthood. As the syndrome never goes away once you have it, by the age of 80 around eight per cent of people have fibro. I suspect my own mother, 88 years old at the time I'm writing this, might have FMS but she doesn't have a diagnosis and frankly she is unlikely to get one because of her age. Age, and its attendant aches and pains, can mask FMS in so far as pain is expected to a degree when old people can't walk, are using walking aids, struggle to open jars, find stairs difficult, and so on. This is especially true when arthritis and rheumatism have been diagnosed. My mother has neither of those but lived with pain for decades before retirement, and, in common with many women of her era, raised her children and put up with a lot. There's arguably not much point at her age, other than for statistics, in diagnosing a condition for which there is no treatment other than what she takes already, namely painkillers. In conversation with her, I've found out she exhibits many symptoms that are hard to pin on anything other than FMS.

We know that FMS isn't communicable - that is to say, you can't catch it from somebody else. It isn't obviously hereditary, either, as mentioned in the previous chapter, although the syndrome can manifest in more than one family member. The chances of you developing it are higher when members of your family already have it. You can, however, find yourself the odd one out with your diagnosis. Nobody else in my own family has a confirmed FMS diagnosis. I only think my mum has it, but can't prove it because I'm not a doctor.

DNA studies of family members (not mine, I'm talking generally) have identified some genes that might explain the tendency, rather than heredity, of FMS to manifest in more than one family member. The genes thought to be related to the development of FMS are involved in how the nervous system responds to pain, with some of them also linked to depression and anxiety. This might shed light on why some antidepressants, such as sertraline, have been found to alleviate symptoms.

If your head is spinning with all the data outlined above, I can't say I'm surprised. Those of us with fibro number in the millions the world over. Focus on that one word: millions. You are not alone if you have it, far from it. And yet, living with this chronic pain condition can make you feel incredibly marginalised, isolated and misunderstood. That results from a combination of general ignorance about this disability among the people we meet, and our realising just how heavily biased society still is towards serving and enabling those who don't have disabilities. Unseen disabilities are even more difficult to get people to understand; there's nothing for them to see. It's frankly difficult, when lying on your back unable to move because of pain, to feel anything other than alone but you can guarantee, whenever you're at your lowest ebb due to the havoc FMS has wreaked upon you, there are countless other people feeling the same way at the same time. All over the world. I don't write that as comfort - how could it be comforting, to know others suffer as you do? - but it is a fact, and we should try to remember it when we do feel alone.

What the statistics don't reveal is the human impact. They don't communicate anything of the misery; the sheer intensity of the pain; the hurt and upset when we encounter people who dismiss our symptoms; the struggle to keep ourselves fed and housed and our bills, including medical invoices, paid. Still, they say that knowledge is power, and this is true. The statistical information helps medical professionals and scientists advance their understanding of FMS. This chapter and the previous one also give you plenty of data to throw at the next smart-arse person who tries to tell you all about the chronic pain condition you live with every day or, worse, seeks to explain it away or paint you as a neurotic fantasist. Your illness is real.

Work, family, friends

A lot of people ask me, "How can you write when you have fibromyalgia?" and the answer is, I write when I can and because, well, I'm a writer. It's what I've wanted to do ever since I was little, not counting my brief dalliance with the idea of becoming an astronaut or cartoonist. I went to college and then university to study with the aim of being a writer in mind. I wrote every day all day after uni, in a succession of high-octane roles, until FMS forced me to stop working full-time because my body simply wouldn't permit me to do the standard nine-to-five (or, as it turned out in the case of the media industry, nine-to-whenever).

The notion of productivity - of being productive - is a very modern one, and a curse on people's health and wellbeing. When we talk of people's productivity, we're referencing them as if they're machines pumping out data, or cloth, or ultraprocessed food. We are all being pushed to do more and more every day. If you're old enough to remember the internet as it was in the early 1990s, you might recall people saying that the advent of email meant the paperless office was just a short step away. Computers, we were told, would take work away from all of us and lead to a society where we had much more free time and a lot less stress. Well. It didn't work out that way, did it?

I remember well enough what full-time work was like before my FMS diagnosis. I worked in the media as a journalist, an editor and as a copywriter for a large corporate publishing house. The work was intense and it never let up. Clients made insane demands, always to be satisfied whatever they asked for, in whatever timeframe, because, well, they were paying the company. What did it matter if the clients were driving employees toward breakdowns? If an employee breaks and leaves the company, you get a new one. Easy!

Friends thought I worked in an industry with an air of excitement about it, even glamour. In reality, I was as much a battery hen as those poor souls in sweat shops on the other side of the world. Better paid, granted, but money can't nullify the impact of stress on the body and mind.

The more brutal in society talk about survival of the fittest, arguing that not everyone working in incredibly stressful situations inevitably suffers a breakdown or the development of chronic illness. To which I'd say, how do they know that? Have they looked at people twenty years after they were working harder than bees and ants? I don't believe high-intensity, high-impact over-employment is good for any worker. Sooner or later, no matter how many times a person says they don't need a social life and are doing okay because they squeeze in half an hour at the gym during lunch, the demands of the modern workplace catch up with the body and punch it in the gut and the head.

When the fibro first hit me full force, my career was effectively killed off. Or so it seemed at the time, when even getting my clothes on every morning had become a struggle that wore me out. I stopped writing because it was tiring to sit in front of a computer, even for half an hour, and the constant banging of keys with my fingers was jarring. This, more than any other aspect of FMS - not the pain, not the fatigue - did me in. I felt I'd been robbed of my ability to do the one thing I had great confidence in, something I enjoyed, the deployment of a skill I'd cultivated for decades. I had two books out - one a novel, the other non-fiction - but it would be five years before I was able to find my way back to writing, and then because of my discovering an aid to writing in the form of voice recognition software. This allowed me to get a first draft done without much use of the keyboard, only subsequent editing and refinements needing me to return to the keys. Still, I had to work around, and with, my FMS. I got to know it well as the years went by, as if it were a person with mood swings. I could write but only when I wasn't suffering badly with my symptoms to the point of being laid flat by them.

Sometimes I can only write for half an hour; other times, for three or four hours, with a lot of breaks of course, more than most people need I'm sure. On too many days I can't write at all, because my hands, my wrists, my elbows all conspire against me with pain to stop me in my tracks. I try not to get down when I'm prevented from writing by my FMS. If I ever let it get me down, under any circumstance, I've found my symptoms seem to get worse. Or at least, they're harder to endure.

There are those for whom FMS puts an end to whatever they were doing with their lives before the onset of the disease/disorder/disability (take your pick). If you are, at the present time, only mildly affected by fibro, it might be possible to continue in your 9 to 5 routine. It's just, with an illness that so often plays havoc with our sleep and makes getting up in the mornings extraordinarily difficult to achieve within a set and short timeframe, people find themselves to have become square pegs trying desperately to fit into the round holes employers expect them to work within. When it starts to get difficult, you can be certain it isn't going to get any easier. Yet people battle on, sometimes causing themselves a great deal of harm in the process. It's easy to understand why: mortgages, utility bills, children, a sense of belonging in the workplace, a shared common purpose. When you reach the point where you can no longer work, perhaps after several periods of extended time off, fear can be as crippling as FMS - the fear of losing everything, ending up homeless, having no real identity when 'all you do' is lie on a bed in pain all day.

As with any disability, FMS shouldn't prevent us from finding meaningful employment, so long as it is flexible and employers are understanding - but that's where the problem is, on the companies' side. They want bright, healthy young things sat behind their desks all day, where they can be seen and monitored, even in this day and age when it is easy to work from home. All too often, working from home is a privilege, a reward reserved for the highest-earning in positions of great responsibility.

Of course it isn't just people with disabilities and long-term health conditions getting the rough end of the stick, it's those over the age of fifty as well. It's more than a shame, it's a shocking waste of people's abilities. The benefits system, certainly in the UK, often doesn't help, piling on the pressure with the underlying question being, 'Are you faking it?' with every phone and face-to-face interrogation. What the constant challenging by the State does is to destroy people's hopes, rob us of what energies we do have and instil immense fear of ending up with no money at all to keep ourselves and our families safely housed and fed.

In Britain, the government says it's doing all it can to help the disabled and sick into work. In reality, maybe not purposefully, it's making recovery and restoration a more distant and difficult to reach prospect. Take, for example, the rule that, if you try to do some work and earn a certain amount only to find that it doesn't work out due to your illness, you're back at square one having to reapply for benefits, prove your illness or disability, and run the gauntlet of hostile actions all over again. Even though benefits are very little, despite what the press might have you believe, when set against a full pay packet, the fear of losing them having tried your best to get back into the workplace is enough to hold people back from trying a job on for size. People too often feel trapped in a sinkhole, unable to find a way back to doing what they want to do. Some compassion and flexibility would go a long, long way.

Government, certainly democratic Western governments, should be about enabling, not disabling; engendering hope, not instilling fear. We might encounter a sea change in policy if only more disabled people got into politics and positions of high office, though we all know the barriers to achievement in politics are as high and insurmountable as they are in the more general workplace.

If you develop FMS and are in full-time employment, it's important to assess your situation with a clear eye. If you tell your employer about your diagnosis, are you likely to receive honest support, lip service to caring or outright hostility? Will you be seen as weak and less able to do what you do, even though you know full well you can still do it, with just a few accommodations? Nobody wants to be chastised or pitied for a health condition, nor do we want people to see us as somehow compromised human beings. We remain human beings, come what may.

"Work is my biggest problem," Sharon, 42, told me. "I was working forty hours a week as a support worker to people with brain injuries acquired through alcoholism, giving them medications, attending appointments with them, helping with cooking and many other things. I've had time off sick due to fibro flare-ups. My boss isn't at all understanding and causes me major anxiety. I had a meeting with her and explained my medications had been increased, that my fibro fog (confusion) was a lot worse. I requested not to give out medications because some of the drugs are dangerous if I were to make a mistake. I broke down, told her how ill I was feeling and how much work was a struggle. She then put me on a zero hours contract because she believed I was going to drop my hours after I said I was applying for PIP [Personal Independence Payment, a UK disability benefit that can be paid to the working and non-working]. It's led to masses of stress about paying rent and other essentials."

It might best serve your interests to hold back on telling an employer for as long as you can, all the while making plans for the possibility of the time approaching when you can no longer work full-time. Some employers, not enough but some, might be in a position to offer more flexible working hours or in other ways accommodate the difficulties you face. To a certain extent, legally speaking, they're supposed to. Still others, like Sharon's boss, could do with acquiring some human compassion and understanding but instead show none whatsoever. If you do encounter unfairness in the workplace, consider calling a disability helpline for advice as this could count as discrimination which is unlawful in the UK and many other countries.

Those with partners bringing in sufficient income might be able to discuss with them the possibility of ending work themselves and relying on the one pay packet. Or, depending on what you do for a living, you could switch to self-employment from home, where you set your own hours and work when you're able, rest when you're unwell.

Some partners are not going to welcome the idea of becoming the sole breadwinner in the household. Others may be more receptive and understanding. If you stop working due to ill health and have a partner living in the same home, the British government provides you with no benefits at all, save for the possibility of jumping through sufficient hoops, metaphorically speaking, to get some form of disability payout. It expects a partner under the same roof to support you, if they earn above a very small amount, whether you've been married twenty years or met your loved one six months ago. This is why the long-term sick and disabled are well advised, if they were single when they first became unable to work, not to move in with anyone they meet and fall in love with thereafter. It's wrong. In the 21st Century, we should all be seen as individuals responsible for our own selves. Nobody should be made responsible for feeding and housing us, save for the State we paid our taxes to until we became too sick to work.

You might, depending on where you stand politically, disagree with everything I've said above. That's okay, but I ask you: in what way is a nation served by marginalising the sick and disabled, driving them into poverty and destitution, making those with partners reliant upon them for survival?

If the time comes that you can no longer work due

to FMS, it's important to seek out advice from disability organisations and neutral advisory bodies such as, in the UK, your local Citizens Advice Bureau. Thanks to the internet, we have access to forums and Facebook groups for those living with FMS, filled with people who will be able to offer you advice based on their own experiences, particularly when it comes to dealing with the interrogatory and punitive benefits system. Seek these communities out, and don't be afraid to ask for help. When it comes to benefit assessments, find out all you can about what's involved in advance of your appointment. Take a friend with you. If you're unhappy with the outcome, appeal it. Many negative decisions are overruled upon appeal.

As well as the economic consequences of being forced to give up work, or having to switch from full- to part-time, there are the psychological ones that can have a devastating impact on your health, including your mental health. Losing work responsibility, almost overnight, can be ruinous to the mind and hazardous to relationships with family and friends.

"Fibro does affect all relationships to a degree," Sharon said to me. "My husband is wonderfully understanding but it does get between us, when he knows I'm hurting or at times when he's afraid of hurting me with touch. We have a 'best friends' kind of marriage and it used to involve play-fighting and doing random silly stuff, which I don't do now for fear of hurting myself. It comes between us when I'm fatigued and he has to do the cooking and cleaning. I feel guilty then, when I see him tired. I get very depressed and closed-off when I'm in a flare."

Guilt is commonly felt by FMS sufferers, as are feelings of inadequacy and uselessness. We can all too easily buy into the idea that we're somehow letting down the human race by being ill and not working. We can end up thinking of ourselves as parasitic. Reject all these and other accusatory self-putdowns that come into your head. They serve no purpose at all other than to make you feel like shit.

You won't get any better by beating yourself up. Plenty of others, wholly ignorant and bigoted, are in this world willing to do that, with no understanding of what it's like to live with FMS and no desire to learn. Don't do what they do for them. Instead, you should always keep in mind words like 'gentle' and 'loving' in relation to yourself. Be kind to you. You don't deserve to be crucified for developing a mysterious and debilitating chronic illness. You're still a worthwhile human being. You always will be.

Similarly, it doesn't serve you or anyone else to worry about the impact of your FMS on those around you, family and friends. True friends will understand, adapt and support. If they don't, they were never really your friends to begin with. Sure, they may be disappointed you have to cancel going places at the last minute - but they can always rearrange with you or switch to calling you up to see how you are on any given day and doing impromptu, rather than pre-planned, things instead. Good friendships are flexible in how they work.

Family is, admittedly, a bit trickier. You choose your friends, you don't choose family. Even so, good, clear communication goes a long way. If you have a supportive partner, take care to show how much you value their support but don't be saying 'sorry' every five minutes. They presumably didn't fall in love with a frequent apologist, so don't become one. Remember, it could easily have been them who found themselves struck down by FMS, or cancer, or some other disease, disability or disorder. We don't know what the future holds. It's fate that determined you ended up in the position you find yourself in. Nobody is to blame, so if you're not to blame for something, why say sorry for it? Saying thank you for help offered, that's one thing, a good thing. Gratitude is essential but don't lay it on too thick.

Explain your illness to your children, if you have any. Children can be far more adaptive and understanding than adults at times. Conversely, depending on upbringing, age and most likely when they are in their teenage years, children can show little to no understanding at all. That's when your patience comes in, I'm afraid, and it's not going to be easy.

There are going to be times when you saying no means no because a request your kids make is wrong or unacceptable to you. Then there are the days when no means no because they're asking things of you that your daily struggle with FMS prevents you from saying yes to.

Your children, like anyone else around you, can and will learn, given time and explanations. Again, good communication is key. Don't try to hide it when you're having a bad day. Say it clearly: I'm having a bad day. In so doing, you give those you love, who love you, the opportunity to avoid asking difficult things of you, to make alternative plans, to be prepared for whatever the day may bring.

Husbands, wives, lovers, children above a certain age, they're all capable of bringing in the washing; vacuuming the living room; making the dinner. Tell them how much their support is appreciated, how even doing little things can be a huge help.

Katy, 35, was a behavioural healthcare assistant on a stroke ward but found herself sweating and struggling to keep up with her co-workers because of her fibro symptoms. Eventually she had to quit. "I found people weren't sympathetic. With fibromyalgia being an invisible illness, they tend to think there's nothing wrong with you."

Katy has an understanding and supportive partner. "He's very understanding of my pain," she told me. "He helps when he can with my daily living. He has mental health issues himself, and ADHD (Attention Deficit Hyperactivity Disorder). Fibromyalgia has never really affected our relationship in any negative way."

Katy considers herself very lucky. Not everyone gets the support they deserve from those they love. Yes, some relationships do fall apart when one partner develops an illness. There's no pussy-footing around the truth: it happens. People split up and get divorced for all sorts of reasons but they can also stick together in extraordinarily difficult circumstances, too. FMS can expose the fault lines in a relationship with a friend or partner, but it doesn't create them. It's sad, but not everyone can handle a partner or friend becoming sick. When friends fall away or a partner takes off, as hard as it is, you need to work on acknowledging you're better off without reluctant, unhelpful people in your life who made a choice not to understand or show compassion.

Many people with FMS find themselves naturally gravitating to others with the same, because of the mutual understanding of how difficult life can be when living with constant pain and the other disabling symptoms.

Kelly is just 21 years old and was diagnosed with fibromyalgia when she was 19. She was diagnosed with CFS (Chronic Fatigue Syndrome) at the age of 13, having had that from the age of 12. Kelly doesn't work because she can't, and quit her last job where she was working twenty-five hours a week. "The manager wasn't very understanding and my situation was dealt with unfairly," she told me. "I quit because they were going to fire me anyway." Her friends are all other people living with FMS. "Some of my family are supportive," she said. "Others, not so much. None of my ex-boyfriends properly understood my illness until I met Jake, who was and is amazing, which is why I married him. He was brought up around illness."

If family isn't what it should be, recognise that family doesn't need to be blood relatives. Family can be whoever. Losing friends is painful but there are so many people in the world who are probably waiting to find a friend in you. Please don't be lonely. Get out there and show the world how magnificent you are.

The things covered in this chapter – work, family, friends – are like the pillars holding up the roof for almost everyone. They go a long way to providing us with a sense of belonging, a context for ourselves. When we can no longer work and lose family and friends because of illness, it can seem like the roof caved in and your life is over. This simply isn't true. It just feels that way.

There's much you can do to help yourself. Be measured in how you approach each day, mindful of what might be too much for you. Try to do a little, gentle exercise every day, when you can. Eat well. Try to socialise at least a few times every month, away from the home, even though the temptation is there to hide away from the world. See if there are any interesting groups local to you that you might be able to join, a creative writing group for example, or maybe a reading group. This way, you can meet new people and get away from those four walls that can seem to pulse and close in on you otherwise. Regular exercise and social activities are good for everyone, not only FMS sufferers, and you might have someone in your life who can take up a new hobby with you. Just don't overdo it, which of course means figuring out for yourself what overdoing it means for you.

You do what you do because you must. Giving up isn't an option you should choose. You do it because you have a right to live your life. You do it because you're a fighter. Maybe you weren't much of a fighter before your FMS diagnosis, maybe you were, but you need to be one if you're not to let this mysterious malady consume your life entirely.

The good news is, we all have the capacity to fight within us. It's part of what makes us human. You need to find that rod of steel inside yourself, seize it and keep going. There are a great many good days ahead of you. Focus on those, not the bad ones. Let the bad ones come and go without holding onto the memories of the pain and fatigue. On the good days you need to build happy memories and a rewarding life. You can do it. I know you can. You know you can.

Restless Legs Syndrome

A syndrome within a syndrome? That's going to sound strange to anyone. Restless Legs Syndrome (RLS, also known as Willis-Ekbom Disease, which is quite a mouthful) is very strange indeed.

There's no evidence that fibromyalgia causes RLS. If you have fibro, it doesn't mean you're also going to suffer from RLS. A lot of us do, though. We either had RLS before we got a FMS diagnosis, or developed it further down the line. People can also develop RLS independently of any other condition, while several other health issues besides fibro are linked to it.

So, what is it?

Well, the first thing to say about Restless Legs Syndrome is: it doesn't, despite the name, only affect the legs. It can affect other limbs as well.

Perhaps it's best at this juncture to detail my own experience. I remember vividly the very first time RLS revealed itself to me. It was several years before I was diagnosed with FMS, and it was a winter evening. I was at home, sitting on the sofa watching TV. Suddenly I started to feel something very odd was happening inside my upper left arm. It felt like an itch I couldn't scratch, only worse than that. It burned like liquid fire. It moved like a snake under my skin, twisting and turning. I've often described it since as feeling like there was too much energy in my arm. It was bursting to get out, like the baby alien in the first Alien movie. It was frightening.

Instinctively, I started to fling or flick my arm around, all over the place. I had to move it. It wouldn't let me keep it still. Imagine, if you will, a burning coil inside one of your limbs, like an electric eel, slipping and curling, this way, that way, every way…

Yeah. You get it. Words like frustrating, agonising, irritating, they don't begin to cover it. I thought I was going mad. I'm almost ashamed to admit, I didn't approach my doctor about it, not for the longest time. When I did finally mention it to my doctor, she didn't hesitate in making her diagnosis of Restless Legs Syndrome. It was new to me but not to the textbooks.

RLS is the biggest nuisance, to put it mildly, when you're trying to sleep at night. It's common for those of us living with it to find the pain either makes it difficult to get to sleep, or wakes us up at intervals, robbing us of precious REM sleep.

When what little sleep you get is in the shallows, it can seriously impact upon your health. Certainly, you can guarantee that a poor night of sleep will make the aches and pains of FMS all the harder to deal with the next day. RLS can strike at any time, night or day. I've even had a couple of occasions when it started to aggravate me on long car journeys, when I was driving. When you're in that situation, your only option is to find somewhere safe to park up and wait it out. An episode of RLS can last just a few minutes to several hours. When you're asleep at night you have no idea what your body might be doing, in terms of movements, but RLS is often found in people who, when asleep, have jerking limbs - Periodic Limb Movements (PLM). If you have a partner, you'll know about this from those times when you've been asleep and have smacked them in the chin or elbowed them in the gut, unaware until they woke you up and told you.

The link between FMS and RLS seems to be an overactive neurological system but, as yet, nobody knows for sure. I've described it at times as 'localised epilepsy'. it isn't epilepsy at all, and isn't linked to epilepsy in any way, but it really does feel like your limb is having a seizure independent of the rest of your body.

RLS, in my experience, doesn't show itself when the affected limb is active. It's always when it's resting. Going back to my story about the car journeys, I drive an automatic and, on a long motorway journey where you can travel for 20, 30, 40 miles or more without turning off anywhere, my hands, and by extension my arms, aren't really doing that much in the way of steering. If other cars, or rather their drivers, are behaving themselves, then such lengthy stretches are at worst boring but you're likely to be somewhat relaxed. Well, I am. I'm alert to what's going on around me, but not stressed - and that's why RLS sometimes strikes me behind the wheel. I can only imagine how much of a nightmare driving at times could potentially be, were it one of my legs, rather than my left arm, tormented by RLS.

When I'm at home watching TV or chilling out with a good book, I'm neither active nor stressed – and that provides RLS with the opportunity, for want of a better word, to strike.

Now, you might say, well then, don't be lazy. But please, come on! Everybody needs and deserves downtime. We all watch TV. A lot of us read. Every living person on the planet has to sleep. What's more, lazy is a horrible word to use against people who find it difficult not only to walk and move about in their daily lives but even find it difficult to open envelopes and tins, to put their clothes on and take them off, to fasten shoelaces and pull socks on and off.

It is vital that people with FMS, whether they suffer from RLS as well or not, get what exercise they can when they can. The recommendation is to do 30 minutes of exercise every day but doctors agree that if you can only do 10 minutes – a short walk for example – it's better than nothing, and it can really help to minimise the incidence of RLS attacks.

You can get RLS in one or more limbs. It most often strikes me in my upper left arm, just below the shoulder but above the elbow. Really, it's quite remarkably specific. I don't know what my left arm did to deserve this, although I am left-handed, which means, I suppose, that my left arm and hand put a lot more work into my daily life than my right. Sometimes I get RLS in both legs and wrists, but never in the day. Always at night. I've been known to run a hot bath at 3am, because I've found it can relieve the pain to a degree. Any relief is welcome. Obviously the very worst thing you can do when RLS strikes is to remain still. Get up. Move about, as best you can. Whichever limb is affected, wave it about. If it's one of your legs or both of them, try dancing on the spot. If it's your arm, or both arms, try doing what I do: fling them about. It's probably best, mind, not to do this with the curtains open and the lights on. You exhibitionist, you. We don't want the men in white coats turning up on your doorstep, responding to a neighbour's concerned call.

Aside from FMS, the risk factors for RLS are many and include pregnancy, sleep apnea, kidney failure, some autoimmune diseases, rheumatoid arthritis, Parkinson's disease, diabetes mellitus, and low iron levels. Something like 20 per cent of RLS cases are due to iron deficiency. If you take an iron supplement, make sure you stop it several days before a colonoscopy otherwise the iron turns the insides of your bowels black. It's harmless but makes it impossible to see if anything is wrong with the tiny camera. I mention this as you're more likely with FMS to end up being advised to have a colonoscopy because of another attendant torment called Irritable Bowel Syndrome (IBS). Doctors often want to know what, if anything, is going on inside you when IBS is severely impacting upon your life. I go into your bowels, as it were, in a later chapter. Won't that be lovely?

RLS is, of course, treatable with medication when frequent and particularly severe. You won't find any pills or potions over-the-counter. You'll have to speak to your doctor. Be aware that some medications, including those you can buy without a prescription, can make RLS worse. These include some antihistamines, antidepressants, antipsychotics, anticonvulsants, and antiemetics. Again, this is why speaking with your doctor about medications is so important. If you're on prescription drugs, and feel the need to buy medicines from a chemist – for a cough or cold, for example – let the pharmacist know what you're already taking before you commit to your purchase. They can advise if it's safe to proceed.

Lifestyle changes help, such as the exercise I mentioned, but also cutting out alcohol and tobacco. In discussion with your doctor, you'll probably hear them reference 'sleep hygiene' as a means to alleviate not only RLS but fibromyalgia as well. Sleep hygiene is common sense, really. It involves such things as not looking at phone and tablet screens for several hours before you go to bed, as well as avoiding tea and coffee from early evening onwards.

RLS impacts upon anywhere between 2.5 and 15 per cent of people living in the United States, and it's not unreasonable to infer the same in other countries. In the UK it's thought to be experienced by up to 10 per cent of the population. Like FMS, it's women who are most commonly affected with RLS becoming much more prevalent with age, although it affects one in five pregnant women in their third trimester. You can get RLS at any age, and in children it's often dismissed as 'growing pains' (there's no evidence growth hurts).

There are two recognised forms of RLS: primary, which has no known cause and starts up slowly before the age of 45, and isn't linked to other conditions, and then there's secondary, which is the sudden onset in association with another medical condition (FMS, I'm looking at you, but you're not the only culprit). Although I developed RLS a few years before my FMS diagnosis, it was secondary RLS, not primary. It didn't start up slowly, I was in my late forties, plus I was already showing other signs of FMS. Certainly, the specialist who gave me my FMS diagnosis saw the RLS as an early symptom.

It is easier to do something about RLS when it hits you than it is to tackle FMS symptoms such as pain and chronic fatigue. You get up, get moving and maybe run yourself that hot bath, even if it's the middle of the night. It's frustrating, really bloody annoying and can be both painful and scary, but at least there are these steps you can take to alleviate it. Far too often with the other symptoms of FMS, you find yourself having to endure them with no way to soften the edges to make life bearable. And that is, as some Americans might say, the absolute pits.

In hot water: hydrotherapy

I've a confession to make: I can't swim. Well, it isn't really a confession, which would suggest I've done something wrong, but it is something I've often been chastised for by family and friends down the years. Why haven't you learned to swim? What if you're on holiday and want to go in the pool? What if there's a flood and you have to swim to safety? You'd drown! These and other questions, some reasonable, some absurd, have been put to me at various times down the years.

I do have experience of almost drowning. I was five years old, my parents occupied with setting up deckchairs on Blackpool beach. They didn't see me go into the sea. I was just paddling, with no intention of going too far, when suddenly the firm sand beneath my feet gave way to nothing. I'd obviously reached a ledge, and gone straight over it. I was swept out by the strong current, some distance from the shore. I still have the memory of that famous landmark, Blackpool Tower, looking tiny in the distance, people like ants or dots. I swallowed water, and went under. More than once. A man rescued me, appearing from nowhere, or so it seemed to me, taking me back to the shore. My parents were frantic by this point, having quickly become aware that I'd disappeared, and they rushed over. There was a crowd of people. Someone told my mum that a man had saved my life. She and my father looked around, to thank the man, but he'd vanished. I don't mean he disappeared into thin air, though who am I to say he didn't? People do believe in angels, after all. I think he didn't want thanks, or a fuss being made of him. The world is full of unsung and anonymous heroes.

I've tried to learn to swim, for the sake of other people, to stop them nagging me, really. Not because I was enthusiastic about giving it a go, as I never was. I had no interest in learning to swim, not because of the Blackpool near-drowning, but ever since I was 10 years old, which was when my teacher thought he was doing good by getting all the children in my class to dive into the pool at the local swimming baths. As I recall the incident, we were supposed to be learning how to swim but there'd been no preliminary explorations in the water, no paddling. We hadn't learned anything beforehand, though some of the kids could already swim by that age. When it came to my turn, I was absolutely terrified and shaking. The teacher noticed this and mocked me. There I was, still only a little boy, with a supposedly responsible adult, an authority figure no less, in truth a total dick of a man I'd never liked and never would after that day, telling me to man up and stop being so soft. Those gender expectations. So, I bit down my terror and jumped in, aware my entire class was watching.

The next thing I knew, my feet slipped on the bottom of the pool and I went under, cracking my head. Even today, over forty years later, I can still remember the sensation of drowning, the panic, my mouth and nose filling with chlorinated water. I must have lost consciousness, because the next thing I knew I was out of the water, at the side of the pool. My teacher had both his hands on my chest, pumping out water. It was well over ten years before I would go anywhere near a swimming pool again. Whenever I've done so, I've always felt that old panic coming back to me. But yes. I did, eventually, try learning to swim again. Several times. I always found it dull at best, completely lacking in joy. For that, I blame that primary school teacher. If we'd had some lessons in how to actually swim before he had us all jumping in, I might have survived the experience, made the dive successfully.

I wouldn't say this childhood incident led to hydrophobia, because I've always loved water. I just don't want to swim in it. Whether I hankered after doing so before my teacher did what he did, I don't know. I can't remember. Maybe what happened at Blackpool had already squashed any desire to learn. One of my favourite things to do today, though, regardless of the season, is to spend time near large bodies of water, such as lakes and reservoirs. I find them peaceful, if having great potential for scaring the shit out of me and ending my life were I to fall into them. After all, I can't swim. If there was nobody else around, I wouldn't stand a chance. I guess that's why I'm always mindful of safety around water, and have a sort of respect for it. I absolutely love the River Thames. I lived, studied and worked in London for 14 years, during which time I'd happily walk for hours alongside that ancient water channel, with or without human or animal company.

I tell you all this as a prologue to the day I found myself getting changed at the hospital into my newly-bought swimming trunks. In conversation with my FMS consultant, I'd agreed to give hydrotherapy a try. I've already mentioned in the previous chapter how both FMS and RLS can be eased somewhat by having a hot bath. Well, think of hydrotherapy as involving a great big bath filled with warm water. At least, that's what I told myself at the time. No, I thought, I'm not really going near a pool for the first time in decades. Should I take along a rubber duck? No. Too much. Just a towel and a bottle of water will do.

You don't need to be a swimmer to give hydrotherapy a go, I'd already been told that, and I was only going to be in the pool for thirty minutes. It was supposed to be the first of several sessions. Note the 'supposed' in that sentence; I'll get to why, bear with me, just not yet. I can't remember the exact number of people who were there, but no more than eight or nine including myself. It was a small pool. I was the only man.

A physiotherapist talked to the group before anyone got in the water, explaining to us what hydrotherapy was, how it might help with our symptoms, how to conduct ourselves in the pool, and what to do afterwards to make sure we stayed safe. It was explained that drinking plenty of water when the session was over was really important, because hydrotherapy can dehydrate you and increase your risk of getting dizzy and falling. The physiotherapist remained on hand throughout the session, explaining exercises and providing support.

So, what is hydrotherapy?

Hydrotherapy is the use of water to treat a number of different conditions, not only FMS but also arthritis and rheumatism. Hydrotherapy doesn't involve swimming (good news for someone like me) but there are special exercises you do in the warm water. It isn't hot, but it's considerably warmer than a typical swimming pool you might attend (unless you're me, because you won't get me into a swimming pool ever again). The temperature is somewhere between 33 and 36°C. It's this heat, combined with the pressure of the water, which is thought to provide benefits.

Don't, whatever you do, equate hydrotherapy with aquarobics – seriously, who comes up with these fitness craze names? – because hydrotherapy isn't anywhere near as demanding as aquarobics. In fact, it isn't strenuous at all. The emphasis is on relaxation and slow, controlled movements. The water supports you, which is great, but sessions are kept short to avoid you overdoing it. You will feel tired afterwards, though, because of the warmth and the mild exercise.

Hydrotherapy isn't like spa therapy. Spa therapy has as its basic premise the idea that minerals in the water work some special magic on you, whereas hydrotherapy is said to be of benefit whether there are minerals in the water or not.

I didn't feel my usual pool panic because the water wasn't deep, and I'm considerably taller now than back when I was ten years old. Actually, I found the whole experience pretty Zen. By the time I got out of the pool, I was feeling proud of myself. As the date of the session had approached, I'd started to feel a little nervous, imagining a great big swimming pool and remembering my dive that was never meant to be, but there I was – not so much conquering my fear as ignoring its siren call to flee, an inner voice that had only shut up when I made my way through the main entrance of the hospital that morning. I guess by that point it knew it wasn't going to win.

My experience of hydrotherapy, the situation and the exercises involved, was positive. Afterwards, as I was getting dressed, I took my first sip from the bottle of water that I'd brought with me. When I was ready, I walked to the hospital café, bought myself a coffee and chilled out for a bit, people-watching. Coffee cup drained, I made my way back to my car and headed home, my bottle of water in the holder between the front seats. I took gulps from it whenever it was safe to do so, at red traffic lights and in the one traffic jam I encountered, caused by a slow-moving tractor.

By the time I pulled the car up outside my house, I'd drunk about half a litre and needed to use the bathroom, which I did, as soon as I got inside. Still mindful of the advice I'd been given, though, when I headed back downstairs, bladder emptied, I decided to have more water and, within about half an hour, had managed another half-litre. So, I thought, I should be sufficiently hydrated by now.

I decided to go for a short walk, my pain levels that day allowing me to do so. It was a moderately warm and sunny afternoon, so the walk was a pleasant one, until I was making my way back home. As I was crossing a busy road, I reached the middle when I suddenly felt faint and dizzy. I had a choice to make, in just seconds: collapse in the road and get hit by a car, no doubt at all that would happen, or try to make it to the other side (by which I mean, of course, the other side of the road, not the afterlife, for which I was not at all ready). As a curtain of blackness descended, I flung myself forward.

Superman makes taking off look so easy.

I must have lost consciousness for moments only. I woke in pain, my face pressed against the pavement, the front of both legs smarting. I was right next to a pharmacy, from which one of the staff came running to see if I was okay. I wasn't okay. Why do people ask that, when they can see for themselves you're anything but okay? I don't want to come across as harsh, because I was truly grateful for the kind woman's assistance in getting me back on my feet. She helped me into the shop and asked me to sit down on a chair. "Just take a little time," she said. "That was quite a fall you had there." I thanked her. I was really shaken up.

As it turned out, my face was covered in cuts and scrapes. I looked like I'd been in a boxing ring, and had lost spectacularly. There was blood all over the front of my jeans, which I discovered when I got home was from a number of cuts and grazes all down my legs. Evidently, despite having drunk plenty of water, the hydrotherapy had done for me. This was the first time in my life I'd had such a spectacular fall, and it was like a preview of old age. I got very little sleep that night, and the following morning my FMS symptoms manifested at their most intense. I could barely move at all, that day and the next.

I suppose it's possible there was another cause for my fainting. I'd eaten before my hydrotherapy session, including something sweet, so I really don't think low blood sugar could have been responsible. I didn't come close to fainting again for several years, and that was when I was in the middle of having a tattoo done, when I hadn't eaten beforehand. Thankfully the tattooist kept a supply of lollipops for such an eventuality, which he told me happens quite a lot. No, sadly, I do think my horrendous fall was down to the hydrotherapy. I just don't know why. The cause can't have been dehydration. If I'd been any more hydrated at the time of my fall, I'd have been a water bed. Nevertheless, I was in no mood to try hydrotherapy again and told my consultant I didn't want to go back for further sessions. I was just too scared after that. Once again, life was telling me, or so it seemed: don't go in the water. For any reason.

In planning this chapter, I was in two minds as to whether to write it at all - or rather, I could have written about hydrotherapy without detailing what happened to me afterwards. I didn't, and still don't, want to put anyone off trying hydrotherapy. Had I not fallen so badly that afternoon, I would have attended more sessions. In the end I decided to tell this story in full because it is my story after all, no one else's. I don't lay claim to any definitive pronouncements on how you should address the agonies of FMS. This is largely an account of my own journey, my experiences with chronic pain, what I've learned. What happened on the day I went for hydrotherapy is very much part of that.

Please, don't be put off. Take this as a cautionary tale. If you do try hydrotherapy, it could be hugely beneficial for you - but don't just take the advice about making sure you don't end up dehydrated, as vital as that is. Had I gone home and simply relaxed for the rest of the day into the evening, I think I would have been okay. I shouldn't have gone for that walk. I spoke with my consultant about it, and they agreed taking it easy until the day after would probably have been a wise move. It's just, nobody actually suggested that to me or the other people attending the session. Advice after the fact is no advice at all. It's hindsight - absolutely useless.

Any course of hydrotherapy on the NHS in the UK has an end date, with you getting maybe three or four sessions. Afterwards you can seek out as many paid-for sessions as you would like. The hospital I attended made its hydrotherapy pool available for paid sessions by prior appointment. If you're a swimmer, or can handle being in the shallow end of your local swimming pool, you can continue your exercises there. Some of these venues have hydrotherapy events, when the water temperature is increased. Sports centres, too, can offer exercise classes in water and some of them don't have daft names like aquarobics, though don't let a name put you off. Check with your doctor, physiotherapist or consultant before you go ahead. Me, I'm sticking with hot baths, and showers when I can handle them. With showers, there are times when the water hitting my body can be painful. That's because of a FMS symptom not every sufferer experiences, called allodynia, which I'll cover in detail in the next chapter.

I don't think I'll ever learn to swim - I don't want to, and that's that - but it's important to state that it's never too late to learn. I'm well aware that swimming is great exercise, both for improving your general fitness and for helping with mobility. If you can't swim and, unlike me, don't have a history of stupid teachers almost drowning you or nearly drowning in the Irish Sea, you've nothing to lose and everything to gain. It might really help you fight the symptoms of FMS and provide you with a new, fun, and highly social activity.

Before ending this chapter, it's worth mentioning another form of water therapy that might be helpful if you suffer from Irritable Bowel Syndrome (IBS) as part of your FMS. It's unproven but harmless, though not easy. It involves downing water soon after you wake up - roughly a litre to a litre-and-a-half, our stomachs varying in size. You'll know when you can't take in any more. For many people, drinking lots of plain water is a difficult challenge even as a one-off. Like hydrotherapy, this comes under the modern day banner of 'alternative medicine' and is referred to as Indian, Chinese or Japanese Water Therapy. Enthusiasts suggest the body adjusts to this daily blast of morning water over time but, at first, it's said it can provoke a significantly increased number of bowel movements, and, of course, more frequent urination.

A number of health benefits are claimed for this type of water therapy. There is a general consensus, among mainstream health professionals, that people in the Western world don't drink enough water and spend much of their time dehydrated. Taking on more water could improve your skin tone, moisturising you from the inside out, and might well alleviate the constipation and pain of IBS while helping to fight the attendant bloating. Don't overdo it, though.

Accidentally drinking too much water is incredibly rare, but upsets the body's normal balance of electrolytes and can be fatal. Water is a poison when excessively drunk within a short time window. And I mean many, many litres of the stuff.

In common with most people, I find I cannot drink water beyond a certain point. I just have to stop. Since developing FMS, though, I do try to make sure I get two litres of plain water down me throughout the course of a day. I've always got a bottle close by, whether I'm indoors or out. I don't drink it because I think it's going to help fight my FMS. I do it because I'm mindful, now that I live with a debilitating chronic illness, that anything I can do in general terms to improve my overall health is a win for me. It's a win for anyone. For me, FMS was the wake-up call that won't switch off. I had to get serious about my health, that was the first thing I thought after getting my diagnosis, although I'd already begun to eat better. I exercise when I can. Just don't ever invite me to go for a swim.

Don't hit me with your rhythm stick: allodynia

Allodynia is the name given to the touch sensitivity and pain many fibromyalgia sufferers experience. It can manifest in all sorts of ways. The water pressure in a shower can be agonising, tucking under a fitted sheet on a bed can be beyond a person's abilities, pulling on socks can take several minutes of wincing. These are just three examples, all of which I have personal experience of, showing just how disruptive allodynia is.

As with any illness, there are tasks and activities you can avoid or find workarounds for. I only wear short sports socks all year round, having long ago had to forsake the type that go all the way up to below the knee. A lot of things in life, however, are impossible to avoid, such as putting on and taking off all your clothes every day. It's also beyond upsetting when the touch of a loved one can make you yelp and draw away from them. The fact that a hug can result in pain coursing through your body results in times when you feel isolated and depressed. We're social creatures, after all. You may or may not be a hugger, but everybody needs to feel the touch of another human being every now and again. Research has even indicated those who receive little to no touch in the form of hugs or other intimacies can lead shorter lives as a consequence.

The effects of allodynia are not constant, some days being better than others, some being a heck of a lot worse than usual. Having to wear more layers and heavier clothes in winter leads to difficulty, while the lighter fabrics of summer provide blessed relief.

The 1979 number one song by the late Ian Dury invited some unknown person to hit him with their rhythm stick, but a well-intentioned slap on the back to offer congratulations for something can leave an allodynia sufferer screaming. Different people describe the pain differently, with some reporting a sort of pins and needles sensation, while others talk of a prickly, intense heat or electric shocks zapping through the affected areas. The sensitivity can be localised or everywhere. The pain can be anything from a mild annoyance through to something that is utterly debilitating. It's thought that sensory neurons cause the pain, and which ones will be different from person to person.

Allodynia doesn't only affect FMS sufferers but also a lot of people with severe migraines, Chronic Fatigue Syndrome (CFS) aka Myalgic Encephalomyelitis (ME), and diabetes.

There are four types of allodynia currently identified, and you can experience one or all of them. The first is tactile allodynia, pain caused by touch. This is perhaps the most common and frequently affecting. Then there is the mechanical form, where pain results from movement across the skin, such as stroking. Static allodynia is a consequence of touch but with the added application of pressure, such as holding hands with someone or another person grabbing your arm. Thermal allodynia occurs when the body is exposed to hot or cold weather and objects, so an ice lolly on the lips might be agonisingly painful or an otherwise lovely summer day.

It's possible there may be at least one more type of allodynia as yet unidentified, because some people report that the use of air fresheners and perfumes in the room they're in immediately provokes a variety of sensory discomforts, such as hands and feet becoming very cold or migraines starting up. People also report apparently allergic responses to makeup, moisturisers, soaps and shampoos accompanying the onset of allodynia, when they had no problems before.

Research into this condition, as with FMS, is ongoing as there's currently no consensus on cause and no known cure. It's thought to accompany FMS because both are said to involve increased sensitivity in the central nervous system. There are lots of medications that have been used to alleviate the pain of allodynia, though some of these are pretty darn scary. They include ketamine, morphine, and tramadol - all addictive and potentially very dangerous drugs.

I don't want to be using any of those, no matter how bad the pain gets. I can understand people accepting the incorporation of these drugs into their daily lives, though, and never say never. Severe pain eats away at our notions of what we will accept, until we reach a point where we have to acknowledge what we need. I just haven't got there yet, and maybe never will. Why do some need stronger pain relief solutions than others? Well, FMS isn't a progressive disease as such, unlike, say, Parkinson's, but when someone has suffered with it for a long time, they're very likely to find themselves becoming habituated to the use of painkillers they were once able to rely on but find less effective as time goes by. I know people with FMS who need morphine patches to even begin to function every day.

Those looking for more natural remedies report the daily use of cannabis or an extract from it known as CBD oil is helpful, although possession of the green herb in many countries if you're caught by the police can result in heavy fines and even imprisonment. I don't sit on the fence when it comes to arguments for and against the legalisation of the use of cannabis for medical reasons. I'm all for it, and the demonisation of a plant that can help people and, even when used recreationally, only makes you laugh a lot and fall asleep, is ridiculous given the extensive harm alcohol, which you can buy all over the place, does to young people every weekend and habitual drinkers and alcoholics all year round.

That said, cannabis can be dangerous to people with severe mental health problems, whether they already take medications or not. And yet it can improve the lives of many with anxiety and depression, so there's a Russian Roulette aspect to the consumption of marijuana that, for many, has them concluding there's too much risk to try it. That's fair enough, given an adverse reaction can impact upon you for the rest of your life. Its availability on prescription, after consultation with doctors and specialists, would go a long way to alleviate worry and ensure the safest possible supply. Regardless, in comparison to drugs like tramadol and morphine, the risk of harm from cannabis is much, much smaller, and its potential for lasting pain relief is real and proven.

Cannabis deserves a chapter of its own in this book, and gets one. The next chapter, though, deals with the topic of sex. Yes, sex. Obviously, allodynia can wreak havoc on your sex life but so too can many of the other symptoms – and medications – associated with FMS. When people talk about safer sex, it's nearly always in the context of HIV prevention, through the use of condoms (yes, allodynia can make rolling those on and taking them off painful) but, in the context of FMS, safer sex isn't only about the prevention of disease but the minimisation of pain as well.

Without further ado, spare your blushes and let's get it on…

Let's talk about sex, baby

Birds do it, bees do it, even educated fleas do it (though where they get the money from to fund their tuition fees, I've no idea). It follows that human beings do it as well - and don't we open up can after can of worms when we talk about sex? Fibromyalgia and sex don't always make good bedfellows.

"I often can't have sex," Debbie, 37, tells me. She's a friend of mine and worked as an administrator in the NHS until she became too unwell to continue, with FMS and progressive rheumatoid arthritis. "My allodynia makes me irritable to the touch. My most recent ex-boyfriend never understood. He often tried to change my mind when I said no. Sometimes it feels like electrical scratching, or I have goosebumps that won't go away. I get extremely short-tempered. My ex-husband found it difficult to fathom what was happening to my body and was convinced I was being 'dramatic'."

Sexual challenges abound for anyone who suffers with chronic pain, FMS being the focus here but there are a number of illnesses and disabilities that routinely have you screaming, shouting or wincing even just putting your shoes on, let alone contemplating sex with another human being. Not only can physical pain inhibit sexual desire and limit the sexual activities available to you, but living with pain every single day of your life and all it assails you with can lead to psychological difficulties new to you since developing fibro. Fear, as we all know, is the worst emotion to feel in any context. Fear - of being hurt in any way - can birth a host of psychologically off-kilter responses when the possibility of taking our clothes off with someone else rears itself up as being on the cards.

It isn't unusual for people living with chronic pain and physically disabling conditions to feel bad about themselves, to feel unloveable and undesirable. Trust me on this: unless your personality stinks and you treat people horribly, nobody is unloveable or undesirable. Nobody. Despair is one of the most devastating feelings that can take root in your mind and heart, but it's sadly all too common.

Negative feelings about your own self and your place in the world, along with a lack of confidence in your sexual abilities, aren't restricted to those of us with FMS or any other disability. Everyone feels crap about these things from time to time. A decent level of self-esteem and positive body image are hard to achieve for the marginalised, the obese, the unhealthy, the rich, the poor, those living with mental health conditions, the short, the tall, the young, the old, the hairy, the bald… Pretty much any member of the human race, in fact. In this age of doctored selfies on Instagram and "Look, my life is fabulous!" posts on Facebook, it's easy to imagine the world is out to get you. It is, when it comes to advertisers wanting to pick at your scabs and make the wounds bigger in order to sell you shit you don't need. People have never been more competitive, even while they're screaming at the world, "I'm not lonely! Look, I have a life! I'm not afraid!"

Life is an insecure ride with no promises or guarantees for any of us. Social media gives us the tools to present invented lives to the world, if that's what we want to do - but the reality, away from the smartphone or computer, persists like a stubborn stain, until you face up to it and look at how you can make things genuinely better. You have to confront the fears that drive you to want the likes on Facebook, the retweets on Twitter. Even if you don't go anywhere near websites like these, the chances are you read newspapers and magazines, watch films and TV shows, get a daily dose of 'you're not good enough, this celebrity is so much more beautiful and successful than you'. It's a load of crap. As is the idea you might entertain in your head that everyone else on the planet is going to be out there having better sex lives and relationships than you can possibly hope for.

Fear provokes the fight or flight response in all animals. In the context of sex, fear can prevent us letting go. It can stop us getting into a sexy situation, reaching orgasm, attaining an erection. Fear presents a less than attractive face to any potential partner. Nobody wants to make love to a person who is afraid, of anything for any reason. Fear is nebulous, hard to pin down. It's smoke and mirrors. Find ways to overcome fear and you can find solutions to problems instead of only worrying about them. You might find the problems were imagined, and don't actually exist.

Sex, in any context, is always about choice, mutual consent, respect, setting boundaries and finding what works for you and your partner. It might be easier for some people to end up in sexual situations than others, but that doesn't mean they're having great sex. Don't mistake 'a lot' for 'worthwhile'. They might be spending all their time between the sheets running away from something inside their own heads. Don't judge your own life by looking at the lives around you, or in magazines or online. And, this is really important, if you're not having sex in your life right now, or you don't even want sex, anyone who says there's something wrong with that is a complete arsehole and needs kicking. Sex is natural but that doesn't mean you have to be at it, or want to be at it. The water flowing off the land on which sheep graze is natural, but I don't want to drink it or I could end up with Lyme's Disease. I'm fairly certain there's something alluded to there but I can't think what... Look, there's no rulebook that says we're required to have sex and partners, nor does any manual dictate the type of sex we enjoy, the frequency, when or where. Plus, no sex is better than bad sex. Being single is better than being with a crappy partner who makes you feel bad about yourself and upsets you.

One of the ways in which you can begin to tackle any fear relating to sexual relationships is to work on not comparing yourself to other people and the world. Being a harsh critic of yourself leads to despondency and feeds the fear you need to banish. Big up the great things about yourself, personality-wise. Whether you've got a great figure or an attractive face is a matter of subjective opinion - if you think you look hot, others might not, if you think you look shit, someone else is going to think you're beautiful. People don't fall in love with bodies, they fall in love with other people.

Fear and worries can be banished with calm thinking, open conversations, trust between partners, and making sure you're in situations where you feel safe to express yourself. They can be addressed by talking, to partners and doctors, and by reaching out for therapeutic help. Psychosexual counsellors ('sex therapists') can assist you in discovering insights into your own self, unlocking mental doors and dismantling walls that prevent you achieving what you want to achieve in the bedroom or wherever you want to get intimate with someone. If you've got it into your head that sex therapists have you getting undressed and doing stuff in front of them, you've been watching top-shelf movies and need to recognise that's a load of nonsense. They are professional, knowledgeable people who can help you without judgement.

I'm going to be discussing 'hookup' apps next, which you can download onto your smartphone. They exist, they're out there, they're widely used. What you or I think of them isn't going to stop people using them and a little knowledge can help people living with FMS decide what is and isn't right or good for them. Ignorance, on the other hand, can lead to upset and danger when people try things without a clue what they're dipping into.

Hookup apps aren't dating apps. Their primary function is to make it easier to meet people for sex. From Grindr to Tinder, they market themselves with phrases like, 'meet interesting people nearby' when, really, most of their users are looking for something more along the lines of fast-food pizza delivery, only male or female with a willingness to disrobe as soon as they get through your front door. If that's not what you want, don't go near these apps. There are others more focused on traditional getting-to-know-you dating.

Hookup apps can be disastrous and utterly devastating for anyone who isn't able-bodied, young and buff, and is looking for something more than just sex. The profiles in these apps generally detail what users are looking for, with an emphasis on physical attributes. Some of them are racist, sexist, ageist and dead set against anyone with a disability or illness approaching them. In the 1960s landlords would routinely put signs saying 'No Coloureds' in their windows to deter people from ethnic minority groups from seeking accommodations with them. Why today we permit people to express what is coyly termed 'personal preference' in such a hugely affronting way on hookup apps is beyond me.

If you try these apps, you have to go into them knowing you might well be rejected by strangers who won't shy away from telling you why they're not interested, and the reasons can be brutal. How would that make you feel? If you can shrug your shoulders and move on to checking out the next profile without getting upset, okay. If bad attitudes expressed towards you are likely to knock your confidence and upset you, then you're potentially facing hurt after hurt after hurt. In which case, don't put yourself through agonies you can easily avoid. You really don't want to come away from these apps feeling worse about yourself. If you do, consider ditching them.

Even if you can get past rejections easily, take great care with regard to personal safety when using hookup apps. Dangerous people can use hookup apps like spiders in the middle of their webs waiting for flies to come along. I'm not being unduly alarmist. There have been news stories I won't go into here, but suffice to say terrible things can happen. Always make sure a friend knows where you're going, and when you get there make sure the person you're meeting knows you've left the address back home with someone.

A big strong person might be able to chuck a stranger out who misbehaves in any way after hooking up online - but can you, when you suffer with FMS? Do you have the physical ability to push someone away who won't take no as meaning no, should you decide to change your mind? You need to think about these questions. Be honest with yourself. Protect yourself. That's my ask of you.

When I wasn't plagued by fibro in my twenties I could easily have considered a one-night-stand. Whether I did or not, that's not your business, but the point I want to make is that there were no physical or psychological barriers to contend with. I had youth, confidence, and agility, but what I didn't have was a chronic pain condition that, at times, makes any movement extremely painful. For that reason, even if I wanted a one-night-stand in the present, I wouldn't. I couldn't.

Imagine a FMS sufferer meeting someone in a bar, going home with this person, doing the whole removal of clothes thing... There's mood lighting, maybe music...

And then...

Owch! Ow! No, it's okay.... I'm just tender... No, I can't do that, my body won't let me... I have fibromyalgia. What's that? Oh, we'll need to stop for a while if you want me to explain... Sorry...

That is not a sexy scenario. At all.

You've just met this person, they want a particular something, you want something too, and you're there saying sorry to them and explaining your pain.

In so many ways, FMS shapes our lives. We have to be aware of this all the time, when people who don't suffer from chronic illness can just go about their business, sexual or otherwise, without any thought given to what their bodies can do, or might do. We often have to talk about our health when we meet people. I'm always watching how I discuss it, what words I use, the tone I deploy, because I don't want to come across inadvertently as being an apologist. I'm not going to say sorry to anyone for my having FMS. No way. The pain is mine, not theirs, so what have I got to apologise for? Nothing.

Physically challenged people do have sex, and they shouldn't apologise for their disability when they're doing it. Wheelchair users do it, people with MS do it, you name the disability and there are people living with it who enjoy satisfying sex lives. It can be done! They don't waste energy on feeling upset and frustrated trying to do things their bodies aren't able to do. They find ways to work around, and with, their disabilities. If, for example, you can't manage the missionary position, you might instead focus on other sexual activities that are comfortable for you. There are many. Side by side, oral and manual stimulation, sexy talk, role playing, massage, to name but a few. There's no guidebook telling you it isn't sex and won't be enjoyable if you can't do it this way or that way. You can take advantage of pain-free or minimal-pain windows of opportunity to get it on, bang a gong and whatever else you want to do.

The romantic route is best for me, a single man right now: proper dating. You meet someone, get to know them, along the way you tell them about your disability. As it's an unseen disability and you don't go out socialising when the pain and fatigue are too much for you, your dating partner isn't likely to have any idea you're living with a chronic illness until you come right out and say it.

"Dating is hard," Debbie told me. "I mean, dating is hard even if you haven't got medical needs. Trying to get a partner to grasp your reality can be nearly impossible."

Chances are, the person you like who's sitting opposite you in the restaurant hasn't heard of FMS. Maybe they'll say their mum or sister or neighbour has it, which doesn't make them an expert but it does at least provide a conversational window into the topic without it all having to be about me, me, me - the realities of your own daily experience. Nothing kills the mood like someone who only talks about their own self, whether it's their illness or their job or whatever. How the other person is going to respond to your revelation is unknown, and that's really scary but it has to happen if you're going to stand any chance at all of building something that has honest, clear communication at the heart of it. If they turn cold and reject you, you had a lucky escape. That's the only way to think about it - choose that way - unless you prefer the idea of being upset long after the bill's been settled and they've gone their own way.

Assuming your disclosure has gone well, you keep learning about each other and enjoying spending time together. Eventually, the big day or night comes when you get intimate beyond kissing. They know exactly what they're in for and so do you. With trust having been cultivated along with good communication, fear and insecurity might not entirely evaporate but they will be considerably diminished.

People who develop FMS while in an established, long-term relationship face their own unique difficulties. Fear, vulnerability and insecurity might be encountered for the first time in the context of getting intimate with a partner. A partner may be understanding, or could display frustration and even anger. Guilt can manifest in both parties. The relationship can come under immense strain, and the commitment two people have to one another might be tested like never before. There may be less sexual activity between you than there was in the past. What sex there is may feel restricted. Your symptoms can stop you enjoying the things you did in the past, or make them more difficult to achieve.

"My sex life is not what it was," Luke, 40, told me. "I find I can lose my sex drive for periods of time, lose interest. When [my partner and I] have some quality time together without the kids, it's very common for me to end up asleep, totally exhausted, or in pain with the fibro. On a good day, if we are together in any sexual activity, the next day I can't move, sometimes straight afterwards, so it's like a burst of energy only to come crashing down. I'm not as active as I used to be."

People change in response to all sorts of situations, and not only is a FMS sufferer going to change but their partner will as well. Whether you manage those changes as a couple, moving forward together into a new relationship configuration, or find you're no longer a good fit for one another - that's up to you. The absolute worst thing a couple can do in this situation is to clam up and not talk about what's happening. If you don't address it candidly with each other, you've every chance of growing apart. Consider going to couple counselling. Talking with a trained professional can give you valuable insight and help with addressing any difficulties you're encountering.

Some of your medications may have a detrimental effect on your ability to become sexually aroused and whether you can achieve erections or orgasms. A lot of the medicines used to treat FMS have their origins in having first been used to treat anxiety and depression. Antidepressants are infamous for having a depressive effect on libido, in both men and women. They can interfere with men's ability to get and maintain erections. Research the side-effects before committing to any new medication regime. It makes good sense. Doctors often don't consider the implications of you taking a drug beyond what it's being prescribed for. They want to make the pain go away but aren't concerned with helping you get it up at the weekend. That's remiss of them. Sex and sexuality are part of the human experience, and you've every right to a sex life. Doctors need to be more holistic in their thinking. If you treat a man's pain but he finds he can no longer enjoy sexual intimacy with his wife, it can lead to relationship breakdown and a deterioration in mental health and wellbeing.

Your doctor might be able to provide you with a drug that counters the sex-depressing aspect of another. Whether you want to get into the whole 'take this drug for that, take this other drug to deal with some of the things the first drug does to you' thing, that's something you need to think about and discuss with the doctor. A good doctor won't dismiss your desire to maintain sexual ability as secondary to addressing your FMS symptoms.

You have the right to seek out sex for its own sake, to not seek out sex at all, to have no interest in it or a lot of interest in it, to cultivate long-term sexual relationships with others, and to work on maintaining established sexual intimacy with your boyfriend, girlfriend, husband or wife. Having FMS does not mean you've signed on a dotted line to relinquish all sexual desire, or passively accept a growing distance between you and a lover as inevitable when it isn't, nor to have the medical professionals you consult see sex as inconsequential if it's actually important to you.

Bad days

When you're hit hard by every symptom fibromyalgia can throw at you, all at the same time, you don't have much option other than to go to bed and stay there. I mean, what else can you do? You can't clean house. You certainly can't go to work. You can't go outside. Even opening an envelope, and I'm most definitely being truthful here, can be a challenge. An envelope! I mean, what? The first-ever day I struggled with one of those was a bad day. I felt ridiculous. A ridiculous man with a ridiculous illness, unable to open the goddamn post when it came through the letterbox. Jar lids often defeat me as well. Pulling up zips and fastening buttons on clothes can be painful. Those metal ring pulls? I ask a friend or I use cutlery to prise them open. Don't even get me started on bath taps. I've had to resort to scissors to open a packet of crisps (potato chips, if you're not British).

The days spent in bed are the worst. I feel lazy, useless, unfocussed and all sorts of other negative things on top of feeling unwell. Bed days are bad days and it's easy to slip into depression over time. Although depression is strongly associated with FMS, it's a consequence, not a symptom. There'd have to be something seriously askew in your mind if you didn't get depressed about your situation. If you suffer from clinical (innate, not dependent on your situation) or situational (external causes exist) depression, you aren't any more or less likely to develop FMS. If you have FMS, though, I find it hard to imagine any sufferer being able to fend off the black dog (as depression is sometimes called) without help from time to time. It's important to talk to your doctor if you do feel depressed. Don't dismiss your own feelings, or think it will lift from you without help.

When you feel forced to retreat back to your bed for days at a time, all you can do is sleep, read books, watch TV - and think. You do a lot of thinking, about your current situation, your past and the terrifying unknown we call the future. A lot of the thinking FMS sufferers do in bed is destructive and makes for the perfect growing medium in which depression blossoms like a dark and poisonous flower. On my own bad bed days, I think of the exercise I'd like to do, the household chores that need to be done, the books I want to write, the fact that I'd like to be out there in the world, socialising, dating, and generally living a life. I think about how much FMS sucks. It really, really does. It isn't just the pain you have to deal with, it's the inactivity forced upon you. Both eat away at the mind. You're like the big tasty cheese and FMS is the hungry mouse.

Four walls become ever more oppressive the longer you stare at them and are contained by them against your will. When an intense fibro flare passes and I'm able to go outside, I'm as excited as a dog when its owner announces it's time for 'walkies'. It's as if I've taken a mood-enhancing drug. I rush around doing stuff, almost manic in my approach, when I should really exercise caution and build up the 'doingness' (yes, that's not a word, I made it up) gradually.

It helps to imagine energy as coins, money in the bank. Some people talk of spoons. They'll say things like, "I've run out of spoons tonight" or "I need to be careful with my spoons today because I'm really going to need them tomorrow". I'm just not one for spoons, really. Not unless I'm using one for ice cream. I talk of energy as money simply because it makes sense to me. I'll know when tomorrow is going to be a bad day because I'll say something like, "I've gone into overdraft, and will have to pay it back". The time spent in bed after exerting myself too much (and what constitutes too much is often hard to discern, because it varies) is me banking energy. Call it recovery time. I envy people who never have to give a thought to managing their energy levels, but that's what anyone with a chronic illness such as FMS has to do.

There have been times when the severity of pain and flare-ups lasting weeks and months have provoked me to say I want to die – or rather, I think it. It's funny, but telling people you want to die really isn't a thing you want to be doing unless you're making a call to a helpline like the Samaritans, who can support you in dealing with the feeling. I really don't want to die, though. Not ever. I've seen death and it's kind of final. What I'm really saying is that I want to live but I want the pain to stop. That's a very different thing.

A line from a song by Robbie Williams often comes to mind when talking to people about the emotional impact of FMS. The song is called 'Feel' and it was a big hit in the UK. The line from it is, 'I don't wanna die but I ain't keen on living either' – and that perfectly outlines the view of many people with FMS. When so much of life is closed off to us due to pain and chronic fatigue, we long for the barriers erected by the illness to be torn down so that we can be free.

When people we encounter in life annoy and frustrate us, we can vocalise our discontent or make excuses to get away (get lost, I have to go see a man about a dog). Online we can block people or mute their posts for a while. With illnesses and disabilities that frustrate us as much as the guy who posts selfies twice a day every day or the woman who insists on talking about her stamp collection all the time, there's no person to shout at or run away from or unfriend online.

So what do we do? Me, I address my FMS like it's a person at times. It's an unthinking, unfeeling thing but I'm not, and I get angry at it. That anger has to go somewhere and I'd rather it didn't get turned on the people I love. I'm not completely mad, at least not yet. I know FMS has no ears with which to hear me, no mind to take in what I'm saying. It won't take offence when I call it names. It just makes me feel a little better to sound off.

The worst thing you can do is bottle up your feelings. If you don't let rip on the fibro, someone you care about might get an earful when they've done nothing wrong. "Come on, you bastard. You're not getting the better of me today," I'll say, when struggling to get out of the bath or a chair. Venting like that helps get me to where I want and need to be, as if the swearing acts like engaging rocket boosters. If you're not a swearer, or there are kids in the house, maybe you can use other words to express your anger and frustration. "By George, you won't get the better of me today, you twisted villain." I really think if you say something like that sentence, though, you should be wearing a monocle and top hat.

Why me? That's the question everyone with FMS will ask from time to time, either of themselves or the universe or the deity they believe in if they believe in one at all. There's no answer to that question. You don't have FMS because someone, somewhere wants to get you. You don't have FMS because you did something awful in a past life. Do you want to swap it for ebola? No, I thought not. We get ill because we're human. Nobody goes from cradle to grave in perfect health until the end comes. What matters is how we respond to illness. The mind has a big part to play. People with FMS sometimes see themselves as being weak but I think the opposite is true. Living with a chronic illness, doing what we can, when we can, defying our symptoms, reveals our strength. Look around your circle of friends, family and acquaintances. I'm sure you'll identify one or two of them you can't imagine putting up with the pain that is your daily reality. Go on. Admit it. Just between you and me. You think your brother or your best friend is really, when push comes to shove, a great big wuss who can fold like paper at the first sign of trouble.

You're not weak. You're a warrior.

When you're at your lowest ebb on a really bad day, you've got to be gentle and kind to yourself. Don't do more than you can and don't feel bad about the things you can't do. If you're capable of running a bath, do so, then relax in it. For as long as you like. On all days, make sure you're eating decent food, not junk. Drink plenty of water. Get outside, if you can manage it, even if it's only into your backyard, and look up at the sky. Notice the clouds, the colours. Get a sense of perspective and context. You live in a big, beautiful world filled with activities, sights and sounds. Breathe, as we all must, but be very much aware of your breathing. Breathing is marvellous. It's an autonomic bodily function, meaning it's involuntary: it just happens. Be in awe of the amazing things your body does and the world around you. Don't beat yourself up. Whatever's going on in your body, you're still in there. Even though it lets you down, it still manages to keep you going.

FMS has led to affirmatory realisations for me, as well as difficulties to overcome. I've learned who my real friends are, the ones who are truly supportive and understanding. I've been able to sort the wheat from the chaff. I've had no regrets about doing that. I've no time for people in my life undermining me, when this disability tries to do that every damn day. I have to deal with FMS but I don't have to deal with the negativity of other people. Conquering my own inclination towards negative thinking is what matters, and I require only good people around me to help me achieve that aim.

I'm glad to have developed a certain clarity as a consequence of living with FMS. I always have to prioritise and work out what's really important for me to pursue, and what I should let fall away. Because I can't work full-time, I've come to appreciate there's more to life than work. When FMS stops you working, though, it can seem as if the world has come to an end. How will you manage? What will you do? These aren't questions we can easily set aside, but life has a habit of bringing us answers when we open ourselves up to finding them. The most common fears in society are of ending up lonely or homeless. We can only address these and other bogeymen by facing them head on and reaching out to others for help. If you don't think you have enough friends, there are a multitude of social groups you can join. If you worry about the roof over your head, maybe you're paying too much for it. Consider downsizing or moving in with others.

When you're not stuck in bed on bad days, there's plenty you can do to occupy your time and prevent your self-worth from disappearing like water vapour from a kettle. Volunteering can really help. Charitable organisations are glad of whatever time you can give them, and generally understanding when you talk to them about what you can and can't do. Okay, you can't climb a ladder in the charity shop to put things on the top shelf, but you can still operate a till and talk to customers. Well, that's great. There's a place for you, somewhere. If you haven't found it yet, keep looking. If you give up, you'll get nowhere, guaranteed.

I hardly wrote anything at all for too many years. I wish I had. So believe me, I know about giving up. I was exhausted, all of the time. I was struggling to cope. And yes, I made excuses and gave in to fear. Fear immobilises you far more effectively than any physical pain can manage to do. It took me a long time to acclimatise to living with FMS. The pain didn't get any easier but my coping mechanisms improved, as did my attitude. Three things led to me writing again, one of them a major life event.

My father died. He was 96 and it was a peaceful death, but it was the fact that I was the only person present with him at the hospital when he died that really impacted upon me - yes, in a positive way even though the loss was devastating. I'd never seen anyone die before. I learned that dying is remarkably easy. It's getting there that can be difficult. In the end, Dad just took a final intake of breath and that was it. There was nothing scary or dramatic about it. In that hospital bed, next to where I was sitting, lay a kind and gentle man who'd been a father to me for over fifty years, had been born before the Great Depression, served with honours during the Second World War, raised five children with my mother, worked the same job for decades and then worked as a cleaner well into his supposed-to-be-retirement years. And he was gone. His body was still there but he wasn't.

I realised, being ill isn't an ending. Death is. The sense of your life being over due to a chronic illness is an illusion. My father taught me many things down the years, and in the end he taught me one of the most valuable lessons of all: seize the day, because it will not come again and you have to make the best of what you've got.

Do what you can, until you can't.

The second thing that got me writing again was buying a new desk. The old one I'd had for years. It was small and cluttered. Books, letters, coffee mugs, ornaments, all sorts of detritus covered it. Most of the time, it wasn't easy to use the keyboard. It was a writer's graveyard, covered in bones. Here lies ability unused. I knew it. I'd known it for a long time. When Dad died, I decided I wasn't going to let FMS hold me back any more. My attitude towards life had to change. I'd been feeling sorry for myself for the longest time but hadn't even been aware of it. I woke up to reality not as I'd fallen into seeing it, which hadn't been reality, but the real thing undisguised by bullshit and excuses. The old desk went for recycling and a new, much bigger one was bought. The old desk had no drawers but the new one had two massive ones, allowing me to keep clutter out of sight and leave the writing space free for writing. I remember looking at my new desk, clear of everything except for my computer, and there, in front of me, was a clarity of mind and purpose made physical.

The third thing that got me back to writing was an aid as useful as a walking stick or handrail. I actively sought out a solution to a problem and found it within minutes of starting to look. This annoyed me, greatly, because I knew I'd used the problem as one of my excuses for inaction. Some realisations can be painfully illuminating. FMS often makes it too painful for me to use a keyboard. I'd allowed this to become my number one excuse for not writing. No more! With a web search that took less than a minute, I found voice recognition software - and immediately cringed at the price tag, because it was far from cheap. £200! I took a deep breath and ordered it.

Buying that software was one of the best decisions of my life. In one effortless (but costly) move, I made my bank account cry but vanquished an aspect of FMS that I'd allowed to put a stop to my ambitions. Alongside the voice recognition software, I bought a top quality microphone because I'd read that relying on the inbuilt microphones of computers wasn't a good idea, and would result in a lot of transcription errors. Sure enough, with the right setup, I achieved 99 per cent accuracy from the word go. The software stopped the pain inflicted on my fingers and hands when using a keyboard - because I didn't need to use a keyboard anywhere near as much, not anymore. Speaking into a microphone is tiring, though. I keep my writing sessions short, and get plenty of rest afterwards. I still have to use a keyboard when a first draft is completed, for editing, but that's okay. That I can manage to do.

Obviously, voice recognition software is great for writers or anyone who needs or wants to spend a lot of time getting words out of their head and into a digital document. It isn't going to help anyone with FMS who was previously working as a carpenter, sculptor or doing some other hand-dependent job, which is most of them. We humans do like showing off what we can achieve with our opposable thumbs. If there's no equivalent to my software solution for the work you used to do, you're forced to ask yourself: what else can I do? I often say writing is the only thing I've ever been good at. It isn't true. I know it isn't. When we think back to our early childhoods, it's rarely the case that our first ambitions in life became what we actually ended up doing. I wanted to be a cartoonist for the longest time. I also wanted to be an astronaut.

Okay, I still want to be an astronaut. But only in a Marvel and DC Comics kind of way, with a cool spaceship.

When you're a child there's an ocean of opportunities ahead of you. As you get older, you can get a sense that there are fewer and fewer avenues available to explore. Yet, there are people with no school qualifications who go to university, for the first time, well into old age. People have terrible accidents and, as a consequence, are forced to switch tracks personally and professionally. A lawyer becomes a painter. A painter might get involved in local politics. A shy person becomes a public speaker. If you're someone who finds your FMS prevents you from doing what you did before the onset of symptoms, you might fool yourself that you've only got one thing in your toolbox and can no longer use it, but that's a way of avoiding tackling the challenge presented to you by fate. I know this all too well, as I've explained.

If you feel stuck, like the FMS has put you on hold, why not volunteer or take a course in something you've long been interested in, photography for example, or creative writing? You don't need to have a grand plan. Just see where you're led by the actions you take. Start by just getting outside and going for a walk, rather than sitting indoors and feeling lost and alone. When you're there, under that big sky, pop into a shop and buy something. Strike up a conversation with the person behind the till. It doesn't have to be deep, just talk about the weather. Or tell someone the dog they're walking is lovely, ask them what breed it is, if it's a boy or a girl. Little things, seemingly inconsequential things, banal things, they all have consequence. They always do. By engaging with the world, we open ourselves up to change entering into our lives and begin to take charge. We also distract ourselves from the pain and fatigue we are experiencing in our bodies. It also helps us when we help others.

Whatever you do, enjoy it. See where it all leads.

Sweet dreams?

People with fibromyalgia have a love/hate relationship with sleep. By that, I mean they love to sleep when they can but absolutely hate the difficulties involved in trying to achieve that blessed state. Most of the time, fibro sufferers describe their sleep as poor and involving multiple interruptions due to pain. How that pain manifests is different in every individual, but the effect is the same: waking up and feeling just as exhausted as when you went to bed, if not more so.

If you don't have FMS, you'll still have had some very bad nights of sleep every now and then. Everybody does. Just imagine every night being like your worst night. Welcome to our world. That is our reality, or it is for over two-thirds of people with fibro. One way of describing the sleep we get is 'non-restorative'. That's textbook-speak. When I have to talk about it in more detail, for example, to a consultant, I go further by saying it's frustrating, involves pain, is horrendously disruptive and depressing.

The thing is, when you don't get decent sleep for a prolonged time, for any reason, you end up walking around like a zombie. You might even start developing a taste for human brains, and jerk your head around like one of the dancers in Michael Jackson's 'Thriller' video. Do I really have to say I'm kidding? You do, though, end up quite a different person to the 'real' you when sleep-deprived. The pains and difficulties experienced during the day are amplified tenfold when you've been woken by your own body countless times during the night. And then there are the times when we get woken up by external factors – pets, husbands, wives, people on the street having an argument right outside your window, police sirens, and so on.

A 2013 study found 61 per cent of men and 32 per cent of women with FMS have a form of sleep apnea, with a variant called Upper Airway Resistance Syndrome prevalent among women. Sleep apnea is the name given to when a person frequently stops breathing while asleep. This can happen hundreds of times in one night. It's dangerous because it means the brain and body might not be getting enough oxygen, and shouldn't be having to deal with a constantly interrupted supply of air. One form of sleep apnea, the most common, involves physical obstruction of the airway; the fault in the second-most common type lies with the brain not sending signals to the body telling it to breathe. Many people find out they have sleep apnea when their partners notice the problem. If you don't have a partner, you're not going to find out whether you have sleep apnea until you raise the concern with your doctor.

In the future, wearable technology could be used to help. A late 2017 study by the health startup Cardiogram and the University of California San Francisco (UCSF) demonstrated that the Apple Watch can detect sleep apnea with 97 per cent accuracy. To do so, it would need to be classed as a medical device subject to regulations and rules it currently isn't held to. Although only the Apple Watch was used in the study, other devices containing similar technology, such as the wristbands produced by Fitbit, could prove equally capable.

There are people living with FMS who find it difficult to get any sleep at all, suffering from insomnia either occasionally or habitually. My own experience of poor sleep is frequent but I only have to deal with insomnia over a period of several days every three months or so. Those for whom insomnia is a nightly occurrence need the urgent help of their doctor to address it, which might involve cognitive behavioural therapy (CBT) and will most certainly involve the introduction of sleep hygiene habits and some form of medication.

CBT involves thinking and talking. It has a proven track record in being successfully applied to a range of health conditions, physical and mental. I've undergone a course of CBT myself. I can honestly say it helped me a great deal with anxiety and countering negative thinking. In conjunction with a qualified therapist, both of you look at your behaviour and thoughts to identify those that are unhelpful, even destructive, to you. You then work on them along with a focus on situations, emotions and actions.

Insomniacs often report that they lie awake in bed worrying and feeling sad, hurt, even angry as they turn over the day's events – and even things from long ago – on a loop inside their heads. Ask someone with insomnia to count sheep, they'll probably start doing so, get to number 47, start thinking about animal welfare issues, switch from sheep to chickens, then think about those poor chickens in tiny cages, what happens to unwanted cockerels... I must confess, that's me. I've long kept pet chickens and advocate better animal welfare to anyone who'll listen. The reason I'm using an example from my own life is to demonstrate that what is worried about is going to be different from person to person, although some topics are going to be fairly common – money, health, relationships and work. You're always going to have worries that are very much your own as well. Like chickens. We all know worrying is a pointless activity. But we do it anyway. We aren't the most logical of beings. Mr Spock in 'Star Trek' is a fictional character, after all (if you didn't know that, I'm sorry to break it to you). While we can all hope to 'live long and prosper', as the pointy-eared sci-fi character would say, we've no chance of achieving a Vulcan-like attitude. A short course of CBT, though, can really help if you're plagued by insomnia and worry. If you're living in the UK it's available through the NHS. Speak with your doctor.

Sleep hygiene is the bracket term used to describe a group of practices and habits that, when applied with discipline to your life on a daily basis, will help you get a better night's rest. I'm really crap at maintaining good sleep hygiene much of the time. I do the best I can, which is all anyone can do, but my best writing times, in terms of how much I can output, are when everyone else is asleep. The world falls silent and there are no distractions. That's the way my creative mind likes it. It doesn't like visitors calling on me, or postal workers ringing the doorbell, or being interrupted in the writing zone by the need to attend a hospital appointment. The huge problem for that mind of mine is, I still need to do stuff in the daytime. I'm especially messed up sleep-wise when I need to get a book out of my head.

Now, wait a second.

Before you start thinking, this guy is about to tell me all about sleep hygiene but doesn't practice it, 'hold your horses' as they say in Lancashire, England. It means pause, and think! Why? Because I made it up. Sorry. Not sorry. I made it up for a reason. It sounded believable, right? Rich in detail - short on truth. I wrote it to demonstrate how all of us make excuses for not getting enough sleep. You will, if you encounter enough writers in your lifetime, come across the excuse I outlined above, many times. It's a load of rubbish. If someone's writing in the middle of the night, it's because they want to do it or they have a pressing deadline and a pay cheque waiting for them upon completion.

The truth is, I write when pain and circumstances allow, always during the day.

Everyone makes excuses for not shutting down or promises things to themselves that they fail to deliver. You might say things like, I'm just going to watch one episode of my favourite show on Netflix before I go to bed. The next thing you know, you've watched five episodes and it's 2am. Or, you're out with friends in the evening and they manage to persuade you to go on from the pub to a new nightclub. Yeah, you've got things to do tomorrow, maybe work, perhaps an appointment, but you'll be okay. That's what you tell yourself. Is it true? No. We want things, we want to do things, and to hell with the consequences - until those consequences hit us. It doesn't help that there's an idea floating around society that people go without sleep when they're busy, active, productive. No. If you can't achieve what needs to be done without skimping on sleep, you're doing too much and need to sort it out or your health will suffer. I don't mean colds and flus that are bad but you get over them. I mean you're risking the development of conditions like FMS that won't go away.

It's time to be brutally honest with yourself. If you want better sleep and less pain, you have to look at changing your behaviour in the four hours before bedtime. Yes. I did say four hours. So, let's get listy (made up a word again) and take a look at what you need to be doing, and what you shouldn't do at all, during those four hours…

Just say no to caffeine, nicotine and booze. You need to avoid these and other stimulants. I'm sorry to be a killjoy but you need to take a long, hard look at what others consider 'in moderation' to be and then dial it down by a factor of ten to get to the level you need to be at.

You might think alcohol gets you to sleep faster, but using it every day, do I really need to spell out the dangers of doing that? Plus, alcohol disrupts sleep later in the night as the body begins to process it, and your liver rightly starts to curse you. Also, be aware that both caffeine and alcohol can pop up in food, with caffeine found in outrageous quantity in so-called 'high-energy' drinks. Please, avoid those drinks completely.

I've never been big on drinking alcohol but I used to drink a lot of coffee. I like my coffee strong. Now I limit myself to 1-2 cups a day. My consultant asked me to consider forsaking coffee forevermore. I told him I needed it to overcome the 'brain fog' that accompanies waking up every morning, particularly after taking amitriptyline the night before. He responded by telling me everyone is an individual and there has to be a little flexibility with the rules, so okay. Look, let's put it this way: if you're drinking three or more cups of coffee every day, cut down. You don't need to go all puritan, unless you want to.

Work that body. Even just ten minutes of exercise in the evening, such as a short walk or cycle, can make a huge difference to the quality of your sleep and your ability to get to sleep in the first place. Ten minutes. It's not a lot, is it? Peel yourself off that sofa, and go for it. Don't try to run a marathon, though. If you do too much exercise - longer than ten minutes or particularly strenuous - it can have the opposite effect to what you're trying to achieve.

Don't get heavy with the food. I'm glad I don't suffer from indigestion very often. It's rare I experience the horrible, burning sensation we often refer to as heartburn. It's not a good idea to consume fizzy drinks and spirits such as gin and whiskey in the evenings. It's also not advisable to eat citrus fruits like oranges or spicy, rich and heavy food or anything high in fat or fried. These aren't going to be well-received by your tummy late in the day. They're guaranteed to haunt you in the night like angry ghosts.

Get outside during the day. Unless you're a vampire or a goth dressed in black cultivating the palest skin possible, you need to get plenty of natural daylight. If you spend your time indoors, your body finds it that much harder to discern night from day.

Resist dealing with someone on the Internet who's wrong. There are billions of people on the Internet, all of the time. At any given moment, millions of those are typing out of their bottoms. I'm not sure how they do that. It must be difficult. Well, you'd think so. The amount of incorrect, ignorant and inflammatory crap that gets posted onto fake news websites, social media and blogs every minute of every day suggests the skill of being able to use a keyboard with your rear end is surprisingly common.

If you're going to take one of these people on, why not take them all on? Because you can't. It's impossible. What's more, where is the benefit to you found in arguing with complete strangers? If you find yourself foaming at the mouth late at night when following a comment thread, chomping at the bit to tell someone how stupid they are and spell it out, point by point, stop it. No good will come of this. All you'll do is get more angry, not less.

As a general rule, people don't win one-to-one arguments on the Internet. If you don't do it first, your opponent will block you. This will only raise your anger to nuclear threat level. Now, imagine, having had a blazing row with someone who lives 3,000 miles away, just before you're due to settle down for the night, what has that encounter done for you? You can be sure of one thing: it's made getting to sleep that much harder. Meanwhile, the idiot across the water will still be an idiot tomorrow. In your view. But hey, I'm not saying you're wrong. Let's not fight about this.

It's just as bad for your chances of getting to sleep if you have a humdinger of an argument with your partner, or anyone face-to-face or on the phone, before bedtime. There's an old saying, 'don't go to sleep on an argument' – and, as old sayings go, it's a good one. It makes sense. It might be that the saying came into being in acknowledgement of the fact that going to sleep on an argument often results in the misunderstanding and division being felt all the more keenly the next morning. It can be so much harder to resolve a dispute if you allow it to roll over to the next day. If you argue shortly before bed, your brain is going to be filled with all sorts of unpleasant electrical and chemical activity. Be nice to your brain. Brains are good. We need brains. Just not in that zombie kind of way.

iDon't with the iPhone. One of the worst habits you can get into at night and even in bed, is using your phone. And by 'using', I don't mean calling people – who does that this century, unless they absolutely have to? I don't mean using one of those cool banana phones from 'The Matrix' films, either. No, I mean staring at the bright screen of a modern smartphone, scrolling through Facebook or watching YouTube videos. I don't know why they call them smartphones, because there seems to be a lot of concern expressed that they're actually making people less smart than we used to be. Something to do with shortening our attention span, making it hard to focus… Oh! Look! A pretty butterfly! Sorry, where was I?

Oh yes. The glow of the screen will severely impact upon your chances of getting a good night's rest. Same goes for iPads, computers, TVs and Android devices. Kindles and other e-readers aren't anywhere near as bad when it comes to affecting your ability to sleep with the exception of the Fire models, which aren't really Kindles at all but multifunctional tablets. You're probably okay with smartwatches, because we look at those momentarily, only glancing at them.

The light your eyes receive from all the attention-grabbing devices whacks what's known as your circadian rhythm completely out of joint. This makes it difficult for anyone to fall asleep and stay asleep. Your brain misinterprets the light as natural daylight, while getting none of the benefits of the real thing. If you can't bear the thought of forsaking all your devices until the morning, most computers, smartphones and tablets allow you to install apps that change the colour hue of the screen from dusk onwards, progressively reducing the impact on your eyes and brain. Some of the names you can search the Web for: Twilight, F.Lux, Iris, Redshift, SunsetScreen. There are others, all capable of doing what you need. Some require a small payment, while others are free. Not all of them have versions suitable for every operating system or device.

If you're reading this book at bedtime on a device with no active light filter, stop it. Please. I promise you, I'll still be here in the morning.

Get comfy. If your bedroom is hot in the summer, you need to open a window and maybe get a fan. If it's autumn or winter and you have the heating on in your house, either turn it off altogether a few hours before bedtime or switch off the radiators in your bedroom. This is because a hot bedroom is not conducive to a great night's sleep. Keep the overhead lights and any lamps low, switching them off altogether when you decide to call it a night.

If your mattress is three to five years old, it might be time to get a new one. People tend to hang onto old mattresses way beyond prime-time. I once had one for an incredible thirteen years! I had no idea how much time had gone by since purchasing it, not until I idly decided one day to think back. As soon as I realised, I ordered a new one. What a difference it made not only to my sleep, but my back as well! An old mattress might, like mine did, look okay and not have any wear-and-tear obvious to your eyes. Believe me, though, when your new one arrives, you'll be amazed what a difference it makes. I know exactly when my current mattress will reach its natural expiration date, as I've put it in my calendar. Synced across all devices, no less. No way am I going longer than five years before I get my next one, although the one I now enjoy is, according to the manufacturer, good for seven years.

Do something nice and do it every night. When you're frequently finding it hard to get to sleep, and/or suffering from the painful sleep interruptions of FMS, your brain and body are confused. Help them out by establishing relaxing nightly routines. Having a nice warm bath half an hour before bedtime can really assist you in getting to sleep, as can reading a book and drinking a herbal tea such as peppermint or chamomile.

People who don't have FMS can be induced to experience the symptoms of it by interrupting their sleep over a period of days. One study involved depriving healthy, middle-aged female volunteers of a full night's sleep by waking them up at intervals for three consecutive nights in a row. The result was they all showed markedly lower tolerance of pain and much greater discomfort and fatigue in their daily lives. Other studies have involved disrupting sleep every night for a week or fortnight, again producing symptoms identical to those experienced by people with FMS.

Much more research needs to be done. The people who took part in the studies presumably got better after a short time, as their bodies caught up with sleep and returned to their normal routines. We don't know how long someone can suffer from interrupted sleep before the resulting symptoms become permanent and diagnosed as FMS. It could vary from person to person. And what other factors are involved? Stress, certainly. Type of employment? Relationship problems? Personality type? Genetics? There are so many potential variables at play. FMS can't be said to be caused by poor sleep, nor can FMS be cured by adopting good sleep hygiene (but you should do it, as it will lessen pain). There is no cure.

It's important to note that the majority of people who are sleep-deprived or have poor quality sleep don't develop FMS but lack of sleep clearly plays a part in developing it nonetheless, for some people. This makes the reality of sleeplessness all the more potentially perilous. Two in five Americans don't get enough sleep at night, by which I mean the recommended seven or more hours. A British survey by the Mental Health Foundation suggested almost one-third of the population suffer from insomnia and 30 per cent would be classed as 'severely sleep deprived'. Poor sleep isn't rare in today's society. It's become an epidemic that needs to be addressed or we will almost certainly see the number of people diagnosed with FMS, mental health issues and other disorders going up as time goes by. So, sleep well tonight, if you can. It's important. If you can't, get to the doctor and ask for help.

Stress

There are people who say fibromyalgia is 'all in your head' - by which they mean it's a psychosomatic disorder, a mental illness with physical symptoms - and some of them are so motivated in their dismissal of the syndrome that they create websites and Facebook pages dedicated to spreading the lie that FMS doesn't exist. What it is that drives them is a mystery but one thing is certain: it isn't a quest for truth. Thankfully, though, real information as to what FMS is and how it manifests is getting through to the general public. Those affected are increasingly vocal and brave, sharing their experiences in person and online. Of course, the pop star Lady Gaga's announcement that she has FMS did more to raise awareness than millions of sufferers around the world could ever hope to achieve themselves as individuals. Such is the age we live in. Many of us looked at the internationally famous singer and wondered how the hell she ever managed punishing world tour schedules and recording sessions when dealing with chronic pain and fatigue. The answer is, of course, Lady Gaga has an entourage of helpers and medics on hand. A person with her wealth and status won't have had to face down disbelieving doctors. Gaga won't have to do the washing up, change and make her own bed, vacuum a house or get kids off to school. How many of us could cope better with the crippling effects of FMS if we were able to afford nannies and cleaners? I don't mean to suggest Lady Gaga has it easy. She has FMS. It's never easy. It's always painful. She's in a position to get the word out, to explain what FMS is, and, to her credit, she does exactly that in interviews. People take notice of a woman who dresses up like a side of bacon.

For all her wealth and privilege, which Lady Gaga wasn't born into as Stefani Germanotta but worked for, I'm sure she suffers like everyone else living with FMS. She's doing incredibly stressful work in a stressful industry, and stress of any kind makes FMS worse. But does FMS ever go away? Well, there have been studies which found 20 per cent to 47 per cent of people diagnosed with FMS no longer met the diagnostic criteria one to two years after their initial diagnosis. I find those percentages very hard to believe. I've never met anyone claiming to have had FMS for just 12-24 months and then that was it, over and done with. I wish. More likely, those involved in these studies entered into a period of remission (when symptoms temporarily subside or disappear). The studies aren't telling the whole story and need follow-ups further down the timeline of each patient involved. What's known is that people who've had FMS for longer than two years are likely to have it for life. I'd be interested to see data on the people involved in those studies after being re-examined, maybe five years later. I'd bet money, albeit not much as I don't have a lot of it, on at least half of them having started to display FMS symptoms again. That's because they're bound to have encountered other health problems and stressful situations in that timeframe - at work, at home, in their relationships. Other illnesses and stress can provoke FMS to flare up.

Stress isn't always bad. If we couldn't feel stress at all, we'd never have made it to the top of the food chain. Not having a 'fight or flight' response would've led to chilled-out cave people getting eaten by sabre-toothed tigers. We've always needed stress, so that our bodies can respond to danger by releasing chemicals into the bloodstream to help us run away from predators. In the modern age, stress helps us stay awake and work hard to meet deadlines or go that extra five minutes on the treadmill at the gym. It can help us argue, defend ourselves and act aggressively. Stress becomes a problem when we experience it frequently or all the time, when it can have a devastating impact on our mental and physical health and sense of wellbeing. If we are already dealing with chronic illness, stress hits us harder.

Stress doesn't result from being chased by prehistoric mammals these days but the causes are many and include lack of sleep, overemployment, underemployment, sickness, being bullied at school or in the workplace, struggling with poverty and debt, relationship problems... These and other stressors affect anyone adversely. FMS can rise up for the very first time, while established sufferers can feel their symptoms are made worse. Take away the stress and the FMS doesn't go away, nor does it immediately calm down. It can take weeks, months, years or might never diminish to any significant degree.

By the time my FMS diagnosis came, at least a decade after I first exhibited some of the symptoms, I was spending most days in agony. I was barely able to move, spending much of my time in bed. I could barely function. I was taking high doses of maximum-strength painkillers every day and amitriptyline every night. I used to make a joke of it, saying I rattled. The truth was, it wasn't funny at all. All the pill-taking combined with the pain and lack of mobility, it made me feel I had no control. I was like a ship lost at sea. The depression was dark and enduring. Then, slowly and painfully, I fought my way back to the world. Exercise, even with the painkillers, was excruciatingly painful but somehow I managed 20 to 30 minutes every other day on the cross-trainer. I began to go for short walks, using my walking stick. I started reducing my dependency on painkillers. The pain didn't go away but I found myself better able to carry the burden of it around with me. My painkiller intake halved and my mobility improved. I reached a stage of living with FMS rather than being entirely caged and ruled by it. It wasn't a perfect situation, far from it. I still wasn't healthy or fit. But it was much better than it had been, and I took that as a win.

Then something traumatic happened, which impacted on me emotionally and physically. As mentioned earlier in the book, my father reached the end of his life.

I'd been living with FMS for almost five years by the time Dad was rushed to hospital for the last time. He passed away two days after Christmas, five weeks after admission. He'd been living in a care home with my mother for eighteen months before that, a situation I'd arranged for them at their request. They'd been living in their own bungalow, a single-story dwelling, for several years before it became too much for them and they needed round-the-clock care. It had to be sold to pay for their stay in a residential home, which broke both their hearts. It was a painful transition from living independently to being dependent upon others. It broke my heart as well. It's a familiar story for millions of children who love their parents the world over.

My parents had granted me power of attorney, which meant I became responsible for managing their lives. My four siblings weren't happy with this at all, perhaps seeing it as being about power and privilege and special treatment. It really wasn't. It was all about duty and having to carry a heavy burden of responsibility. I'd agreed to take on stress. I don't know how I managed. I did, though. I handled all the bureaucracy, the decisions that needed to be made, the forms that needed to be filled out, the long car journeys back-and-forth, the hospital visits, the meetings with social workers and medical staff...

All the time this was going on, I expected my FMS symptoms to flare up like a gas fire turned up high. But no, with a little help from friends and a few more painkillers, I got everything done. Looking back, I know my parents and I lived through a prolonged period of extreme crisis and seismic change. Inside me, there was this person who was utterly exhausted and screaming in pain. I ignored him, something that would ultimately prove destructive. I sidelined agony, storing it away in box after box in the attic of my mind, knowing full well that those boxes would eventually overturn, the contents spilling out to give me hell.

Not yet, I thought. Keep it together…. Keep going… Keep fighting…

I had stressful arguments with my brothers and sisters during that transition period. Every decision I made, which my parents had expected me to make on my own as they didn't want care by family committee, was challenged. In the end, it got so bad I blocked emails and phone numbers, contacting my siblings only when I had information I felt duty- and conscience-bound to impart. I'd never been close to them – I was born fifteen years after Number Four, twenty years after Number One - but their behaviour when Mum and Dad went into care permanently severed what little connection there'd been between us. They could have helped out but chose to be obstructive instead. They visited the care home every four or five weeks but never took our parents out anywhere, socially or to hospital appointments. That was all left to me, and their visits never lasted longer than an hour. They missed out, I believe. I got to know my father better than ever before during his eighteen months in the care home. The time we spent together I'll forever be grateful for.

When I was little, Dad worked long hours and I didn't see much of him. I knew he loved me. One of my most enduring childhood memories is of him, dressed in his black workcoat, resting his bicycle against the back wall of the house. I can still see my comics, rolled up, in his pocket. He bought them for me every week, collecting them from the newsagent. When the first issue of the 'Star Wars' comic came out, Dad went round all the shops in my hometown looking for a copy. From my teenage years on, though, my father and I struggled to understand and connect with each other. It was only when he entered the care home that we rediscovered our connection, and talked.

My father knew I had FMS but never understood it. He suffered from vascular dementia in the last seven years of his life, a long time to live with that condition, but he remained capable of conversation right the way through to just a few days before he died. He'd greet me whenever I visited the care home, which was three or four times every week, and ask, "Are you not well today?" This was his way of acknowledging I was living with a strange malady that caused me pain. "I'm all right, Dad," was my reply, always, whether true or not. He'd have worried himself sick otherwise. I couldn't do that to him. Still, he was canny and able to read faces. He knew when I wasn't being truthful. I think he knew why.

Dad's final admission to hospital was because of a lung infection, not his first. He suffered from Chronic Obstructive Pulmonary Disorder (COPD), a dreadful consequence of having smoked from the age of fourteen up until he was 50. For at least fifteen years before he died, he coughed up phlegm many times during the day and night. He'd often get chest infections, which were treated with antibiotics - lots of antibiotics, their potency increasing over time. This time, though, after two weeks of antibiotics in the hospital, Dad was sitting up and looking much better. His nurses told me the infection had responded well to the antibiotics, and they began talking of how to facilitate him leaving the hospital. He was in a weakened state, so they were considering a nursing rather than residential home. It would have meant separation from his wife for the first time in almost 70 years. Both my parents were distressed at the prospect, my father unable to entertain the idea at all, my mother resigned to its inevitability.

It wasn't to be.

Dad contracted an antibiotic-resistant strain of E. coli, which took up residency in his bowel. A doctor sat down with my mother and myself, informing us that an antibiotic mix of last resort was being tried. We were told if there was no improvement after five days, there was nothing more that could be done. During those five days, every time we visited my father, we looked for signs of recovery. By the end of that time window, we already knew before the doctor spoke with us, from our own observations, that the antibiotics hadn't worked. I was holding it together well, all things considered, until I asked, "How long does he have?" and was told four to five days. The infection would quickly spread now from my dad's bowel to his chest, and blood. Then I cried.

My father stayed eight days before leaving us. His passing was peaceful. I was the only other person in the room. I'd lost my best friend to lymphatic cancer the year before, but hadn't been present when she died. From the moment of Dad's death right the way through organising his funeral and wake, I did everything that was needed and required of me with calm and determination. If I felt any FMS pain and fatigue at all, it was ignored. I can't honestly tell you if I had any symptoms while Dad was in hospital or during the three weeks after he died up to his funeral. In all likelihood I probably did, but everything was put on the back burner. I functioned. I remember some of the well-intentioned comments. You're doing so well… You're being strong for your mother… I think you're doing an incredible job… It wasn't a job. I was arranging my father's burial. I didn't have to be strong for my mother. She was and is the strongest person I know. Was I doing well? I didn't have a clue.

I was glad when the wake was over. I went home and collapsed, feeling more exhausted than I'd ever felt throughout my illness.

I slept for twelve hours.

I didn't wake up refreshed. It was the longest uninterrupted period of sleep I'd had since I was a teenager. Pain was coursing through my body. I felt wretched. My grief had come to the fore and my FMS fed upon that grief, running riot through every part of me. Even my fingertips hurt. My toes. The FMS was back at full intensity with a vengeance. All the stress, physical and emotional, which I'd held back somehow in order to do what needed to be done, it broke through and washed over me now like a tsunami. It knocked me on my back. The only way to respond to it was to listen to my body, and rest.

If you suffer the loss of a loved one and have FMS, you can expect your symptoms to get worse for a time. We have to move through our bereavement in much the same way we cope with pain: we put one foot in front of another, and keep going until we start to feel better. There's no shortcut through grief. When someone dies it's like a big rock has been thrown into a lake, and there are ripples from it which take time to disappear.

"My mum was terminally ill, then passed away," Sharon disclosed to me. "This was a huge stress trigger for me because I lived an hour away by car but don't drive. I relied on people giving me lifts. I think not knowing how long she had, and worrying she would pass without me, that was a big trigger as well."

When something as stressful as the death of someone close to you knocks you down, it's understandable if you want to be a hermit and hide away from the world but it's not going to be good for you to do that for very long. If you're stuck in bed, call a friend. You never know, they might have a story to tell that will make you laugh. Laughter is no cure but it does make you feel better. Just listening to another person and them listening to you can diminish pain and make you feel that little bit brighter. If you're able to get up and go out, even if it's the last thing you feel like doing, do it. Even if it's only a short trip to the shops and then home again.

I was invited to a friend's birthday party in a nightclub, not long after my father died. I really didn't want to go - too soon, too much, not feeling it, in physical and emotional pain - but I found myself booking a hotel room and buying new clothes, even though every fibre of my being was screaming I should stay at home. My mood wasn't upbeat or sociable. I didn't want to be around people. But you know what? When the day arrived and I got to the venue, there I was, listening to music and being dazzled by the lights. I got into conversations with people I knew well and some I didn't know at all. I was glad I made the effort. I felt a little bit better just by being there, in the company of others, somewhere other than inside my own home.

Although stressful life events are nearly always going to be accompanied by an increase in the severity of FMS symptoms, there are things you can do to help yourself that don't really require a lot of active thinking when you're likely running on autopilot much of the time. Keep moving, try to eat at least some decent food, drink plenty of water, rest when you can and get as much sleep as you can. Be social, even if only for brief periods on the phone rather than in person, letting friends and family know you're hanging on in there. Don't let other people add to your stress levels. Remember: bad and good days alike come to an end when you go to bed and turn off the light.

The cannabis conundrum

We generally see plants as benign, with the exceptions of those that are poisonous or carnivorous (not that any of them eat people but instead slowly dissolve insects). Yet among all the hydrangeas, tulips, roses, dandelions, nettles and more - flowers and weeds - there is one species of plant that has, through no fault of its own, attracted more controversy than any other: cannabis, an annual flowering herb.

You can smoke cannabis, drink it in a tea, use it in baking. It's also known as marijuana, cannabis being its Latin name. It can land you in jail, depending upon where you live in the world. In the UK, growing cannabis or being found in possession of large amounts of it can land you in prison for years. But what, you might ask, has this got to do with fibromyalgia? The answer is pain relief.

The cannabis plant has been found to have many beneficial pain-relieving properties. It's the fact that cannabis is used recreationally which has resulted in it having a shady reputation. It's hard for me to understand why. I mean, when used solely for pleasure like alcoholic drinks, the usual effect of cannabis is to make people exceptionally chatty, laugh a lot and, if enough has been smoked or eaten, fall asleep. This is in stark contrast to the effects of alcohol intoxication, which I'm sure we all know include aggression, vomiting, becoming stupidly argumentative, verbally and physically abusing strangers, and collapsing unconscious. Alcohol is notoriously addictive. There's no proof that cannabis is physically addictive at all. People like it and go back for more, but report no ill effects when they abruptly stop taking it. Alcoholics, on the other hand, can't just stop without medical support. If they never stop drinking, the chances are they'll not only die from liver or other organ failures but they'll have destroyed their relationships and careers before getting there.

The UK government rejects calls for cannabis legalisation and regulation, and claims a substantial body of evidence shows consuming the plant to be damaging to both mental and physical health. It sticks to this line like a broken record, flying in the face of evidence provided by scientific research and people who appreciate the pain relief cannabis provides. Meanwhile, countless legal and prescribable drugs can be harmful if used for long periods of time and all have their share of possible side-effects. Take opioids, for example – a family of drugs used by millions the world over.

The truth is, cannabis can be harmful to people with mental health problems. The fact that the drug is only obtained illegally means you take your chances, when and if you decide to try it for the first time. Kind of like Russian roulette, you don't know what's going to happen. If cannabis were legal, however, you'd be able to obtain it from your doctor after consultation. If it wasn't suitable as a means of addressing your health problems, your doctor wouldn't prescribe it. If it was appropriate for you, you'd go away with your prescription to the chemist and collect your medicine. The people at risk of cannabis proving hazardous for them would know.

This seems the sensible approach to me. Legalisation would remove risk by involving doctors in prescribing, and put an end to criminal gangs making millions of pounds. That money would go to the Treasury instead. Would there still be an illegal market for cannabis? Undoubtedly, but then there is an illegal market for most prescription drugs. The size of that market would be tiny compared to the black market that operates today.

There's no doubt in my mind, after reading and talking with people about their experiences, that cannabis has the potential to do a great deal more good than it can ever do harm.

The pharmaceutical industry has a great deal of money to lose if the number of opioid prescriptions were drastically reduced by marijuana take-up. Data from the US, where some states have legalised medical marijuana, shows this is exactly what happens. In those states, between 2010 and 2015, prescriptions for opioids dropped by 2.11 million daily doses a year when cannabis was legalised for medical use. When dispensaries opened for the drug, the drop was 3.7 million daily doses. That's one study. Another, using data from 2011 to 2016, found states with medical marijuana laws saw a 5.8 per cent reduction in opioid prescriptions, while those states with recreational cannabis laws saw a 6.3 per cent drop. Both studies appeared in the Journal of the American Medical Association internal Medicine, and generated a great deal of media interest worldwide.

What's the problem with opioids? Well, they're highly effective for pain relief but prolonged use makes them less so. People end up taking more than they once did, to achieve the same effect. As with heroin (itself an opioid) and cocaine, the dosage just goes up and up if it's to provide the same relief (when it comes to medical use of opioids) or hit (when used recreationally).

In the US alone, in just one year (2016) 64,000 people died from overdosing on opioid painkillers. One of the most famous victims was the pop-rock star, Prince, who, by the time of his death, was suffering from immense hip pain. His death resulted from an accidental overdose of fentanyl, an opioid many times more powerful than heroin. Opioids legally prescribed for pain relief include morphine, hydrocodone, oxycodone and methadone. These are hugely dangerous drugs when taken in doses higher than those your doctor advises you to take. Sadly, when someone with severe pain has a prescription bottle of opioid painkillers to hand, it's all too easy to take another tablet if your agony hasn't been relieved by your usual dose. It isn't stupidity. It's desperation.

I was once listening to an interview on BBC Radio 4. A doctor was being interviewed. It was a while ago and I've forgotten the context, but I remember the doctor saying there was no reason why, in Britain today, anyone should have to live with pain. The doctor went on to advise that those of us in severe pain should speak to our GPs. There's always something a doctor can do, that was the message - and it simply isn't true. Yes, a doctor can prescribe pain relief. No, that pain relief isn't always sufficient. It doesn't matter how many times you see your doctor, there are only so many pain-relieving drugs available to prescribe and so many pills you can safely take each day. If you max out, you're out of luck. Chronic pain sufferers often describe their pills as only 'taking the edge off' the pain they experience.

I've got a powerful representational image in my mind. There's a person with FMS standing alone. A doctor nearby throws them a pill and they catch it with their tongue. The doctor then throws two pills. Again, the fibro sufferer catches and swallows them. Next it's three pills. Then four. It's getting harder for this person to catch all the tablets and swallow them. Still, they try. Five. Six. Seven. The number of pills just goes up and up. Eventually the poor soul is buried under a mountain of tablets. You can't excavate them from their predicament because to do so could kill them. You ask if they feel any better, and the answer? No, not really. Maybe a little.

FMS sufferers often start out on standard over-the-counter pain relief such as aspirin and paracetamol, before diagnosis. When diagnosed, they might get prescriptions for low-dose codeine at first, only slightly stronger than the stuff they can buy without prescription. After several years of increasing dosages and ever-stronger pills, they might end up being prescribed morphine patches. In the absence of alternatives and with pain needing to be alleviated, what choice do they have? FMS affects people in many different ways. Pain is always subjective. We each experience it but none of us can convey how it feels. We just know we want it to stop. In the absence of a cure, doctors can only throw pills our way and those pills become less effective over time.

Instead of the person buried under a mountain of pills, let's imagine another scenario. Again, there's a person with FMS standing alone. A doctor, close by, hands over a seed. The person plants the seed and it grows into a cannabis plant. They eat a leaf and feel better. The doctor, twiddling thumbs, has nothing to do. After a while, the fibro sufferer feels pain returning, so eats another leaf. At some point, the doctor decides to take the plant away. While not very happy about this, because the pain will return, the person with FMS has no withdrawal symptoms. If they don't get their plant back, though, they're likely to start considering pain-relieving alternatives that are highly addictive, nausea-inducing, constipating, indigestion-causing – and legal.

I've no idea if a single fresh marijuana leaf would do anything at all for anyone. I'm just using it to demonstrate my argument, which is that prescribed cannabis, when compared to opioid painkillers, is going to be considerably gentler. If you could get a prescription for cannabis, your chances of overdosing would be zero. It cannot kill you. If you are one of those at risk of harm should you consume cannabis, your doctor wouldn't prescribe it to you in the first place.

Instead we have a situation where sick and disabled people are criminalised, maybe even imprisoned, if they seek out something that works for them and is illegal, while those that don't want to do anything illegal (understandably enough) continue to suffer. This is the cannabis conundrum. I cannot, in good conscience and with a strong sense of responsibility, ever recommend anyone break any law for any reason. I can, however, advocate for change to the law because, in my opinion, where a humble plant is concerned, the law is an ass. The general public remains divided by views that are either ardently pro or vehemently anti, with 47 per cent supporting the sale of the drug in licenced shops.

Katy is in favour of cannabis legalisation. "I smoke it quite regularly and it does help with my pain but mostly it helps me sleep. Cannabis use carries a stigma, though, so I don't tend to tell people about using it as a form of pain management."

Sharon was introduced to cannabis a year after her FMS diagnosis. "The pain was unbearable and I wasn't coping well. A friend told me about CBD oil and I invested in a CBD vape juice [e-liquid for use with e-cigarettes]. I found it took the edge off the pain. The same friend gave me a little bit of cannabis to try, and I've never looked back. The relief it gives me is immense, and immediate. I feel like me again for a while. If I was able to grow cannabis and not get into trouble, I definitely would as I think I'd have a reasonably normal life."

Kelly is neither for nor against the use of cannabis for medicinal purposes. "I've heard lots of people say it helps with the pain but, after seeing the effects it had on my druggy ex-partner, I'm reluctant to use it myself."

Luke believes the low-dose CBD oil currently legally available in the UK is overhyped. "I personally found it useless. I'd go so far as to say it's a placebo. Over the years I've smoked and eaten cannabis but don't see any point to legalising it as I see no obvious health benefits."

Change is coming. A cannabis-based medicine has been licensed for use in the UK only recently. The drug is called Sativex, or nabiximols. It's a spray administered orally that contains two extracts from the cannabis plant. One of these, delta-9 tetrahydrocannabinol is more commonly referred to by its acronym, THC. THC is the component of the marijuana plant responsible for it having gained notoriety as much as popularity. It's the stuff that gets you high. You might read in the papers about the other ingredient of Sativex, cannabidiol (CBD). Incorrectly, the media often references CBD as being the pain-relieving chemical in the plant, while THC is the 'trippy one'. THC also relieves pain, though, at least as effectively as CBD. Some THC users claim it to be significantly better than CBD when it comes to addressing FMS pain and fatigue. Sativex is only available for the treatment of spasticity related to Multiple Sclerosis, for now. You cannot get it without a prescription and it can't be prescribed to alleviate FMS symptoms.

Sprays containing only CBD in a vegetable oil are legal to buy, and have become widely available without prescription. CBD can also be bought in pills, vaping fluids (for e-cigarettes, containing no nicotine), drinkable liquids and skin creams. None of these products can ever result in intoxication. You're safe to drive and go about your business. If you're using something with CBD in it and find yourself talking a lot or laughing, that's you. It isn't the drug. I found CBD oil, administered orally with just a few sprays several times a day, allowed me to cut back on my use of prescription painkillers. I told my doctor and she was all for it. The NHS could not only save a lot of money were medical cannabis to be legalised and made much more widely available, but it would undoubtedly save lives.

Marijuana has a long and somewhat fascinating history. There are entire books written about it, and so only so much I can squeeze into a single chapter. It has been used as a medicine for at least 5,000 years. There are hundreds, if not thousands, of different strains. Inevitably in the modern technological age, ways have been found to increase the THC component for those wanting to get ever more intoxicated. The drug as it presents on the streets, in compressed block form, as dried buds and, less frequently, as oil, can be contaminated by other substances. These can be harmful to varying degrees. It follows that legalisation, with attendant oversight to monitor purity and quality as well as distribution, would reduce risk overnight.

In 2014 my friend Debbie's neurology consultant stopped her using Tramadol and codeine. "I overused them, for migraines," she explained to me. "I ended up hospitalised at one point." Within days of her access to these drugs being cut off, she was in agony. "I couldn't move or even put on a bra," she said. It was then that another friend of hers mentioned 'wacky backy' – a term used in the UK to describe cannabis. "My nan used to call it that," said Debbie.

As she had a four-month wait until her next appointment to see a rheumatologist, Debbie decided to try cannabis for herself. "I started by baking it. I made brownies. I'd have one small square a night, and it helped. It lessened the stabbing pains and electrical waves I'd get disrupting my sleep. On rare occasions, I'd have maybe five or six puffs on a spliff [a joint, a cigarette containing tobacco and cannabis]. That was when the pain on a scale of one to 10 was way beyond 10. I found it really helped me get back some control over the pain in my body."

I asked Debbie if she had any regrets about making the decision to try cannabis. "Without it," she answered, "I'd have been sat in a corner rocking back and forth. My consultant has since put me on morphine patches to control my pain, but to be honest they just take the edge off. I'd much prefer, and hope for, the choice of having NHS-prescribed marijuana patches instead of opioids."

Debbie's story isn't unusual, in that many people who are prescribed strong painkillers accidentally overdose on them. She was lucky it resulted in a hospital admission she didn't come away from in a box, and she knows that. Her introduction to cannabis wasn't unusual either. With it being a hot topic of conversation in society, cannabis is often suggested to chronic pain sufferers by their friends, who aren't always up on the law and just want to be helpful. Some of those friends know someone who knows someone who knows someone else, which is how people end up sourcing cannabis in sheer desperation for something - anything - to alleviate their suffering. Debbie is far from the stereotypical image of a pot-smoking layabout teenager listening to music in their room all day. She's in her late thirties, a single mother to two children, neither of whom are ever exposed to seeing their mum using cannabis for pain relief.

A man I'll call Michael used cannabis recreationally in his student days. "It was a long time ago," he said to me. "I didn't go near it again for at least a decade, not until I got a fibromyalgia diagnosis and not even then, not for a long while." Michael decided to take up cannabis again when he became concerned about the effect opioid-based painkillers were having on his stomach. "I couldn't take them without having a full stomach," he explained. "Even then, I had terrible stomach pain afterwards. Resulting from what I was taking to help with the fibromyalgia pain! It made no sense to me. I'd often have terrible indigestion and soreness that wouldn't go away for ages. I just decided one day: I'm sick of this."

Michael sourced cannabis in the form of dried buds, which, as a smoker already, he used in joints. "I'd forgotten how to make them. When I got the hang of it again, I found I didn't make them as strong as when I was a student. I didn't have more than one, either. Always at night before bed. My days of getting absolutely wrecked were behind me." Did Michael find his symptoms improved? "Yes. Not only did I stop feeling like my guts were being stripped, but the fibromyalgia pains were much relieved. Better than with the painkillers my doctor gave me. I found especially that I could get to sleep at night, and stay asleep."

Michael doesn't now smoke. "I gave up about six months into using cannabis every day to relieve my pain." He now uses an electronic vaporiser, which gives him a way to burn cannabis leaf without use of tobacco. "It's clean. I'm not getting nicotine or the other rubbish in tobacco, and I only need to put a little bit in the device to get enough of a dose to do the job of relieving my pain."

Cannabis will, eventually, be legalised. The question is when. It could be decades away. Until then, the cannabis conundrum remains something only each individual living with chronic pain can address for themselves. Whatever decision you reach, be careful with those opioid-based painkillers. Don't increase your dosage without first getting approval for doing so from your doctor and, if they say no, ask for some other form of pain relief from them. A drug called Naltrexone is one possibility, not something I've taken myself, but it's referred to as an anti-opioid, used to treat addiction to opiate-based drugs. It also treats some autoimmune diseases, and has shown promise in treating the pains associated with FMS. It's not clear how it helps, although it's thought it might work as an anti-inflammatory acting upon the central nervous system. The dosage is low but there can be side-effects including a temporary worsening of symptoms and many of the problems associated, ironically, with opiate usage: sleep disturbance, diarrhoea, constipation and stomach pain. These can be alleviated and do stop within a short timeframe.

One person dying from opiate accidental overdose is too many, and there are thousands dying every year. Don't be one of them.

Pains in the backside

Backside, bottom, arse, booty, ass, bum… We use so many words to describe our back ends, yet we're as reluctant to talk about them when things go wrong as we imagine the Victorians were about anything at all going on under their clothes. Maybe it's down to us associating our bums with unpleasantness, given what comes out of them. Or perhaps, when there are worrying symptoms back there, we get scared because we can't see for ourselves what might be wrong. We experience the pain, and sometimes see problems in our stools. Beyond that, we are quite literally in the dark.

If you have any problems going to the toilet, or see blood in your poo, it's really important to make an appointment to see your doctor as quickly as possible. Whatever is going on, they can help.

The most terrifying prospect of all is, of course, bowel cancer. Early identification of the disease increases your chances of beating it. Over 41,200 people get a bowel cancer diagnosis every year in the UK alone, with more than nine out of ten cases being discovered in people who are over the age of 50. Over 2,500 new diagnoses made annually are in people under the age of 50. If you have fibromyalgia, you're no more or less likely to develop bowel cancer than the general population but it's not at all uncommon to find you have a different, non-fatal but often crippling bowel complaint known as Irritable Bowel Syndrome (IBS).

How they relate to one another is not understood, but FMS and IBS appear strongly linked. Over half of those suffering from IBS also display symptoms of fibro. It's thought the two conditions can impact upon you at the same time, flaring up together, or independently of one another. The pains of FMS tend to be in the skin, muscles and joints. IBS pain is inside the bowel. Working together in an unholy alliance, the two conditions provoke debilitating fatigue and despair. They prevent or make difficult social interactions, and can drive even the most outgoing person into seclusion.

IBS involves food moving too quickly or too slowly through the digestive system. Normally, the large intestine makes food pass through your system with rhythmic muscular contractions. With

IBS, the work your large intestine does is somehow disrupted. This results in a number of difficult symptoms, which include:

Diarrhoea and/or constipation. The inability to pass a normal stool is one of the most frustrating aspects of IBS. It doesn't matter how healthy your diet is, how much fibre you take in, the result in terms of what comes out of you is always going to be unpredictable. You can suffer diarrhoea one day and constipation the next, or encounter both within a few hours of each other.

When you're suffering from constipation, it's important not to strain (push hard). Doing so increases pressure in the bowel and is thought to be one of the factors leading to the development of diverticular disease, where pouches form in the lower intestine and can become infected (diverticulitis). Diarrhoea is obviously not going to be difficult to get out of you, but can still involve a lot of pain in its passing.

Bloating and wind. Bloating affects IBS sufferers at any time. I find it tends to happen in the evenings with me but there's no fixed rule. I start the day with a flat stomach, knowing that by around 9pm the belt on my jeans is going to be cutting into me due to the expansion that takes place. I notice it when driving for long periods as well. I start out comfortable and flat-stomached, only to eventually find myself having to unfasten my belt when traffic lights are on red, because the discomfort is extreme otherwise.

You can call it vanity not to want to look like I'm the world's first male pregnancy when I'm out with my friends, but I'd disagree. My build is reasonably slim and I'm not overweight. Bloating doesn't make me look fat, it just makes me look strange with this bulbous lump in front of me. I'm conscious of that. It does nothing for my confidence. You can say nobody notices until the cows come home. I don't care. I notice. That's enough. And whatever your normal size, bloating isn't just unsightly. It involves discomfort and pain.

During the day when I know I'm going to be socialising at night, I avoid foods that encourage bloating and gas, such as legumes (beans, chickpeas, lentils and peanuts, to name but a few). I drink lots of water. Carbonated drinks are out. Bread is a no-no. I consume foods I think are unlikely to irritate or scrub my insides, such as light soups. Watching what you eat helps. It's not a guaranteed fix.

Wind can emerge at both ends when you're alone or in company. Whether it stinks like somebody died or not, the sound alone can have you wishing the floor would open up and eat you. It's a product of fermentation in the gut and, like bloating, can be addressed to some degree by what you eat and drink. If there's nobody else around apart from a cat or dog to judge you, I wouldn't be too worried. Again, if you're going out and will be spending time in the company of other humans, you might want to do as I do and watch what you eat beforehand. If food or drink contains or will provoke gas, avoid it.

One thing I've found helps in fighting gas and bloating is taking probiotic supplements, such as acidophilus. Plain, natural yoghurt also contains these and other so-called 'friendly' bacteria. Everybody has a mix of 'good' and 'bad' bacteria passing through and living in their digestive system at any given moment; it's thought those of us with IBS might have an imbalance, where the bad bacteria far outweigh the good. There are no side-effects to 'topping up' your good bacteria, just as long as you stick to the dosage on the label where capsules are concerned. If you do take too many in one go, you'll probably get the runs for a little while. You can eat as much yoghurt as you like.

Exercise is very good at dislodging trapped gas, so it's no bad thing to suggest going for a short run several hours before a night out. It might be a good way to minimise the risk of embarrassment that would accompany blowing a small hole in the side of a restaurant or club. Eating quickly, which many people do, is known to provoke gas. Eat slowly and make sure you chew your food. Avoid chewing gum, as this gets plenty of air into your system to wreak havoc later. Smoking and vaping also draw air into the digestive system. You might have food and drink intolerances which compound the problem, and it's worth keeping a journal to track when you have the worst issues with bloating and gas. You'll then hopefully be able to identify food and drink causing gastric disturbance.

Stress plays a part in worsening and provoking bloating and gas. It follows that relaxation, meditation and rest can all help minimise the problems you encounter. Don't forget your doctor can help, by recommending lifestyle and dietary changes, and prescribing medicines that will alleviate your suffering.

Diarrhoea, constipation, bloating and gas are the most common IBS symptoms, but mucus in stools, frequent bouts of acid reflux (indigestion) and a general feeling of nausea are also frequently reported. A particularly bad episode of either constipation or diarrhoea or both in fairly quick succession, one after the other and then back again, can result in a feeling of being absolutely drained like you've run a marathon. And, in a way, that's kind of what your bowel has done when you're in that situation.

Drugs prescribed to treat IBS include antispasmodics (which reduce the twisting and turning in your gut), laxatives to address constipation or anti-motility drugs to fight diarrhoea. Check with your doctor before trying any natural remedies. Some of them, particularly activated charcoal, have the potential to interfere with your body's take-up of medicines prescribed to manage your other symptoms. Medicines prescribed to treat FMS also have the potential to exacerbate your problems with IBS. Opioid-based painkillers, for example, are well-known for causing constipation.

Somewhere between 10 per cent and 20 per cent of people living in Western societies are said to suffer from IBS at some point in their lives. It can come and go, although if you have FMS along with IBS, the IBS is pretty much a constant companion – manageable but always there.

Because I've never been able to see what's going on inside me, and none of us ever can, it's impossible to say when my IBS morphed into diverticular disease. I reported to my doctor that my IBS symptoms had reached a whole new level of intensity, the agony reducing me to tears and completely disabling me for weeks on end. I described it as 'IBS++' and was prescribed a bowel analgesic, which made the pain endurable until I was able to attend for a colonoscopy and a gastroscopy, both booked on the same day. The results of these showed inflammation in my oesophagus suggesting food intolerances, and diverticula (pouches) in my lower bowel.

The specialist recommended I avoid gluten in the first instance in response to what was going on in my oesophagus. I'd already found out for myself that going gluten-free significantly reduced my bloating and digestive distress. I was told that coeliac disease (a lifelong autoimmune disease caused by a reaction to gluten) and gluten intolerance are found in a lot of FMS sufferers. I'll cover gluten in more detail in the later chapter on food and drink.

The cause of the diverticula was something of a mystery. They aren't uncommon but tend to develop as you get older. Only one in 20 people have them by the age of 40 but over 50 per cent of the population has them by the age of 80. Nobody knows why some people have them and some don't, although Western diets lacking in fibre and high in salt, sugar and fat are thought to increase the chances of them developing.

I'd been eating a high-fibre, healthy, vegetarian diet for well over twenty years prior to the diverticular disease diagnosis, ever since I got out of the bad habit of eating quick, convenient rubbish in my student days. I didn't think I was a likely candidate for developing diverticular disease but later found out the diverticula might have formed in response to my taking a steroid, Prednisone, for four years. It had been mistakenly prescribed as a treatment for my FMS. It and other steroids, taken over long periods of time, can weaken the lining of the bowel and make the development of diverticular disease more likely.

Causality is impossible to prove, though. I already knew the steroid overuse had led to me developing osteopenia (a weakening of the bones making me more likely to break them if I fall, not necessarily a precursor to osteoporosis but requiring a daily calcium supplement). Thanks to the osteopenia, I lost an inch in height. I'm tall and went from 6'2" to 6'1". I could bear the loss, but still... It was upsetting. There was no way to recover my height. It was gone. I joked - at least I think I was joking - that I never got the chance to say goodbye to that disappeared inch of mine. In all seriousness, though, prescription errors are common and can have these and other appalling consequences.

People with FMS are no more likely to develop diverticular disease than the general population. I mention it here not only because it's part of my story, but because there's no way of knowing if you have diverticula or not until you have a colonoscopy. You can have diverticula present for decades and not know. When diverticular disease does manifest, it's indistinguishable from IBS save for it being a lot more intense and prolonged when it's giving you grief. They share the symptoms of bloating, diarrhoea, constipation, pain and nausea. Diverticular disease can develop into diverticulitis, which is when the diverticula become infected. This is a serious condition that involves high temperatures and a general malaise with extreme pain and vomiting. Treatment involves a liquid-only diet to rest the bowel, and antibiotics. If a person often suffers from diverticulitis - gets infections repeatedly – then surgery might be proposed to remove the affected part of the colon. That is extremely rare, though.

If you've had IBS for a long time, doctors will often recommend, in their efforts to get to the bottom of it (pun intended), that you undergo a colonoscopy. The prospect of it can be daunting, but really the worst part is the clearing of the bowel by use of prescribed laxatives the day before the procedure. They're not driving a bus up there, after all. It's an incredibly tiny camera. You can be sedated if you're particularly nervous. I asked for sedation when I had mine, but it wasn't the colonoscopy that worried me, it was the gastroscopy. I was really worried about choking, though the specialist told me that doesn't happen, ever. After the fact, I can say both procedures weren't difficult experiences at all. I wouldn't have known I have diverticular disease and food intolerances without these explorations.

Don't be reticent about talking to your doctor if you're having any problems with what's happening inside your bowels and at your rear end when you go to the toilet. Men seem especially reluctant to drop their trousers in front of medical professionals and undergo rectal examinations. It's why so many men needlessly die of prostate cancer. As a man, I don't understand it at all. Maintaining your health and getting treatment for whatever ails you, these are far more important than a misplaced sense of impropriety or notions of bodily invasion. For goodness' sake, let doctors examine you properly and give you the help you need. We all, male and female alike, only have one body. When it stops working, that's it. Pain inside the body, as a rule, doesn't just go away on its own. It's a sign. It's the body's way of telling you there's something wrong.

There's always something that can be done to make you feel better - dietary changes, lifestyle changes, medications. You can alleviate symptoms, even if you're stuck with a condition for life. Your bottom is as much an essential part of you as every other organ in your body. You ignore problems at your peril. So don't.

Get away from the negatives

The sacrifices we make and losses we're hit with on our journey with chronic pain, the people and things we have to give up, are many. These are the burdens and emotional punches not touched upon in news reports about fibromyalgia. They aren't symptoms. Living with FMS we can be surprised and distressed to find out some people choose not to understand and even go out of their way to make life more difficult for us. They can be close friends and family.

I once wrote my siblings a letter, like a Dear God letter, never having any intention to send it because that was not the point. I wrote it to get my feelings and thoughts out of my head, onto paper. If you're finding anyone in your life challenging and frustrating, and don't feel able to let it all out to them and get anything other than hassle in response, I recommend doing this. You sit down, clear your head as best as you can, and write your letter knowing that afterwards you'll put it in an envelope, seal it, and stick it in a drawer. It can be tremendously cathartic. It doesn't matter who you're writing your letter to - father, mother, siblings, best friend, former best friend, ex-partner - as they'll never see it. Them seeing it isn't the point of it. You're writing to help yourself, providing an outlet for an aspect of yourself desperate to be acknowledged. Your spelling and grammar can be awful - it doesn't matter. You're not writing to win any awards or make sales.

In my letter to my brothers and sisters, I wrote that, 'You are the worst brothers and sisters I could ever have hoped not to have'. In that one sentence, I condensed a lifetime of being misunderstood, maligned and hurt. All too often, anything that happened to me in my life was greeted with a collective shrug by my siblings and a general attitude of not giving a damn. When they learned of my FMS diagnosis, one of them might well have gone online to look it up, only to come away from websites somehow having managed to take the facts and distort them. It's a thing that women get... Oh, it's all in his head... He just had to get a strange illness, didn't he? He's workshy, that's it...

How can I be so certain of what they would say, how they would react? Because time and again, over half a century, I became all too familiar with how their minds worked in relation to anything to do with their youngest brother. From before I could even walk, indeed crawl, they'd begun as teenagers to form opinions of me. I think they were jealous of a baby. My parents did their best to shield me as I grew up, and they intervened on occasions, but when you're dealing with four against one, well, it's not going to prove that successful. You can't watch all the time and you won't see everything. And you won't change the underlying attitudes, either.

When I developed FMS I found any ability I had acquired to cope with my siblings' pettiness and odd rivalry evaporated. Because I live with chronic pain, I avoid conflict wherever possible and prefer to walk away. My zero tolerance approach is consistent whether I'm having a good or bad day. On bad days, I'm too focused on getting through them to pay any attention to the dramas people create around themselves for attention and controversy. On good days I want to enjoy being pain-free while it lasts, knowing tomorrow might be horrendous. The last thing I want to do, when I'm able to do all the things I really do want to do, is embroil myself in stupid arguments face-to-face or online. Those with disabilities both visible and invisible are keenly aware that life is too short to be dealing with other people's shit.

When I cut my siblings out of my life, limiting my exposure only to necessary notifications, I removed the source of emotional pain that had been ongoing throughout my life and could flare up, just like the FMS, at any moment for any reason. I've done the same with other people: cut them out and moved on. I'm aware this makes me sound brutal but I'm really not at all. I remain the person I like being: sensitive, intelligent, caring and creative. I have many faults, of course, none of them uncaring or vile. I'm imperfect and unfinished, just like everyone else and I'm okay with that.

Cutting pain-inflicting people out of your life prevents them from doing any new harm but you still have the past to address if you want to fully heal and not be influenced in the here and now by things that may have happened decades ago. Therapy – talking to a counsellor – has helped me enormously. The National Health Service in the UK provides very little in the way of talking therapies, a short course and that's it. Yet talking to a counsellor, knowing it's in confidence, can be beneficial to many people in helping them work through their issues, past histories and behaviours. If you can afford to pay a private therapist, there's no limit to the number of sessions you can have. A good therapist will never tell you what to do. They will listen and ask questions designed to help you find the answers within yourself. That's one of the strange and wonderful things about human beings: we can have questions worrying us, going round and round in our heads, often for years, when the answers to them are also inside.

We all have personal histories that are far from perfect. If you have a fantastic relationship with all your blood relatives, I'm pleased for you but I don't waste time on envy of anyone with regard to any circumstance. Envy, like worry, is pointless and self-defeating. The truth is, even if your family isn't dysfunctional, throughout your life you're guaranteed to encounter horrible people and situations. They say how you respond to them can be the making of you, that tough experiences make us stronger. I'm not sure that's entirely true. I think it's a nice idea but the reality is that stressful, negative encounters can be bad for our health and general well-being.

We learn but we don't always learn the best lessons. Someone who's suffered abuse, for example, might have learned to stay away from people, isolating themselves. I certainly did, for a time, when my relationship of fourteen years ended suddenly. I hardly wrote a thing for almost five years. For the first two of those years I spent a lot of time on my own, largely by choice. When our responses to pain, be it emotional or physical, prove limiting and self-defeating, that's when therapy can be at least as helpful, if not more so, than certain medications. Often it's a combination of therapy and medication that gets you through difficult times. When depression isn't clinical, it's situational, meaning external factors are pressing upon you. Pills will alleviate the feeling and help you live your life but therapy addresses the causes of the feeling. Even money worries. It won't bring you money but it can help you find ways forward out of debt.

When we develop FMS, we live with the symptoms for quite some time before a name is put to them. For some of us, that can be a matter of months but for many it's more like years. Just because we don't yet know what's wrong with us doesn't mean we aren't ill, although there are people who won't accept the symptoms of others as real and valid until a doctor has made a declaration as to what is actually going on. It's strange. Stranger still is the fact that people routinely challenge the diagnoses received by others. When my mum was diagnosed with delirium after an operation, one of my brothers and a sister were convinced she had Alzheimer's.

For the most part, the years spent with my ex-partner were good, even great. There were always problems to overcome. It's the same in any relationship. We did overcome them, until I began to exhibit symptoms such as chronic fatigue. At first, I didn't apply too much thought to what might be happening. Neither of us did. I was simply exhausted, a lot of the time. I don't recall the day when things started to change between us. All I know is, the putdowns began. There was nothing wrong with me. I was being 'unbelievably lazy'. I wasn't 'pulling my weight'. I was 'good for nothing any more'.

The illness hadn't driven me to my doctor yet, let alone a rheumatology specialist to confirm a diagnosis. I didn't know what was wrong. I started to believe the things I was being told about myself. Having them repeated to me, day after day, night after night, drove the negatives deep into my mind. I couldn't associate tiredness, exhaustion, with illness. I thought of being unwell as involving symptoms such as coughing, sneezing, catching a vomiting bug, having a strange rash, getting the runs... Now, looking back, I know my grasp of what constitutes sickness and disability was limited.

My ex wasn't aware of being abusive. My ex was frustrated and angry. There was no malign knowingness behind the constant drip feed of negative statements about me, no sense of the damage being inflicted. I didn't know I was being abused, either. Most of the time, what was being said made sense to me. I had no alternative answer as to why I would spend a day wilted on the sofa, nor why I would put off routine household chores like vacuuming. I was confused, suffering from the brain fog common to fibro sufferers, not knowing why my head was so muddy. It was only after the relationship ended, when I was out of the house and living in a place entirely on my own, that I phoned a helpline and let it all out. The man I spoke to was in no doubt at all when he said I'd suffered sustained psychological abuse. He told me it would take some time to move beyond it, and he was right. It did.

'A Pain That I'm Used To' is a song by rock band Depeche Mode, and those suffering from any form of abuse, over a prolonged period of time, do get used to it. I ended the relationship by saying no. My ex delivered an ultimatum I rejected. I was ordered to go after a job I knew my symptoms wouldn't let me do. If I didn't, I was told, we were over. "Then we're over," I said. By the time your partner is ordering you to do something or else, any love in the relationship has disappeared like steam from a kettle.

I had no sense of the damage being inflicted by the constant stress, arguments and negative statements made about myself as if they were facts. The attacks made against me because of my illness were making my illness worse. As with all chronic illnesses and invisible disabilities, FMS can make a person feel terribly alone. Add to that the loneliness that comes from being in a loveless, critical, lop-sided relationship, and the recipe terrorises you almost to the point of paralysis. To say I was scared of living on my own after all that time spent with another person would be an understatement. I knew physical strength and endurance had leeched away from me, that I wasn't as capable as I'd once been. I felt as vulnerable as a chicken cornered by a fox.

I remember well the day I left the home we had made together. A very dear friend was with me, watching as I popped the key through the letterbox once all my things had been moved out. She held me as I dissolved into tears. The new place I'd found for myself had recently been renovated throughout, and felt immediately welcoming when first viewed. Still, I didn't know how I'd manage, what I'd do. With all my boxes of possessions around me and my friend having gone home, I realised something and it was, I think, the start of my fightback: with my front door closed and locked, my new house was quiet. There would be no fighting there, no arguments, nobody making me feel bad about myself. I made myself a coffee and sat on the sofa, fussing the cats (my ex hadn't wanted any of our pets, telling me they could go to a sanctuary). I told my feline friends everything would be okay, and think they might even have understood.

Men find it difficult to talk about pain. Generally speaking, it takes them much longer than women to even tell anyone they're suffering, let alone approach a doctor for help. Too often men are raised to conceal emotion and limit their sharing. It's even harder for them to seek out help when on the receiving end of abuse in a relationship.

Men stay in relationships in which they are being abused for many of the same reasons as women: they are frightened, feel ashamed, have children to protect, suffer from low self-worth, have religious beliefs playing a role, and they might be in denial. In addition, when they're in a same-sex relationship, men might not have come out to family and friends, and fear being outed. There are fewer resources for men suffering abuse, with some encountering disbelief from authorities or having the impact of their abuse minimised because they're male. Some people even believe men are naturally violent and should therefore be able to take control of situations and defend themselves. Bullshit.

It's my hope, having written about my experience, that any reader, male or female, in a bruising relationship will know they are far from alone and go get the help they need and deserve. If you have FMS, that's the only pain you can't escape from and have to learn to live with. What you don't have to accept is anyone making you feel worthless, adding to your pain emotionally and physically. You are better on your own than with somebody who's bad for you.

I cannot overstate how important it is to have only positive, supportive people in your life when you struggle with FMS every day. You cannot make people understand - you can't make people do anything - but you sure as hell don't have to put up with a lack of understanding and anyone sending negativity your way. If you do put up with it, that's a choice you've made and will have to live with until you decide to change the situation. I tell you now, though, you're not helping yourself at all. When dealing with a fibro flare, pain coursing throughout your body, peace and quiet and absolutely no hassle from anybody else are essential to getting through it.

In my many conversations with other chronic pain sufferers, I've found one thing we have in common is the ability to feel bad about ourselves and the situations we are in. It's destructive and pointless but we've all been there from time to time. The corrosive effect of FMS on our mental well-being is real, and has to be fought and addressed alongside the physical symptoms. Let me make this clear: you didn't cause your FMS. No action of yours, no lifestyle choice, no career decision, no perceived personality flaw, no, none of these things made FMS come upon you like a visitation from a dark angel. Your door wasn't marked. You didn't invite it in like a possessive spirit into a willing host.

As hard and unfair as it is, you just got ill.

Given this inclination we commonly share to beat ourselves up, the last thing we need is to accept others doing that as well. If they won't change, you have to walk. As for how you see yourself, stop looking in a funfair crazy mirror and take a look at your real reflection. That's a human being deserving of respect, love and kindness, right there. I don't care what your background is, you can stop thinking bad thoughts about yourself and get rid of the people who are bad for you.

My life got so much better after negative people stopped playing starring roles in it. I started writing again, began to socialise and made new friends. I'd never go back. I have no regrets. Most days, even when I'm feeling pain from head to toe, I'm generally happy because I captain my own ship and have built up both my confidence and self-worth.

If your life isn't good right now, it can and will improve if you take the necessary actions to cut out the dead wood. Your symptoms won't go away but you'll find you do more with your life than just cope and endure. Without other people's issues getting under your skin, you'll find yourself. Change starts by wanting it. So want it.

Matters of the mind

Your mental health will suffer with any prolonged illness. How could it not? When you consider the impacts of fibromyalgia symptoms such as chronic fatigue and severe systemic pain, how could they not bring you down? Everyday tiredness can make all of us a bit short-tempered in conversation, but round-the-clock exhaustion is more likely to have those suffering from it hiding away from any form of social interaction at all. Impaired mobility and cognition (the ability to think, understand information and follow conversational threads) appear, at first, to be much easier to cope with when home alone. When there, you can choose not to move if it's going to hurt you and conversations don't happen unless you count addressing your pets. You can easily avoid answering the door or picking up the telephone. The truth is, being home alone can become a health issue in itself. Isolation makes us more likely to develop new mental health problems and make established difficulties much worse. We're hardwired to be social animals.

If you have FMS, I don't need to tell you how emotionally, psychologically, physically, socially and economically devastating it often is. If you don't have it, believe me when I tell you it's all of these things.

"My mental health has suffered because of my rheumatism and fibro," my friend Debbie divulged to me. "I've felt unwanted and useless. It's hard to get out of that destructive mindset, especially when ex-partners or current throw snide remarks at you when you're vulnerable. Then it becomes easier to believe, oh, they must be right, look at me! I tell myself to stop it, that I'm strong. With the pain I deal with every day, not even the world's best CIA or MI5 operative could cope with that level of sustained torture."

The person living with fibro has strength, there's no doubt about it, to be able to get through every day. It's not a strength that comes from muscular capability but from the mind and heart. Because most people equate strength with physical capability, those of us with FMS are too often seen as weak or, even more horribly, lazy. We are neither of those but we sometimes think we are, because everyone is being pushed to do more - work longer hours, sleep less, go to the gym for two hours after work, work, work, work...

What do you mean, you slept? How self-indulgent.

Look, sleep is necessary. Work should not be anyone's entire life. How did we get to this place? This super-bionic work ethic, if you can call it an ethic at all, is everywhere. It's fit for robots, not people. It oppresses anyone who can't do everything they're asked to do and more – and that means everyone is oppressed, sooner or later, because not even the greatest athletes are capable of running marathons for their entire lives. And there's a price to pay. The battle to simply live, to avoid being overwhelmed, can cost all of us dearly, not only people with chronic health conditions, and our mental health gets impacted upon by what we go through.

More than half – 56 per cent – of fibro sufferers are also fighting anxiety, while 62 per cent develop clinical depression in their lifetime. I've had anxiety and depression to deal with on and off down the years, and these are commonly experienced by people from all walks of life, rich and poor. One in four people in the UK alone experience a mental health problem every year. They don't all develop FMS, nor did they all have FMS before they had issues of the mind to contend with. What FMS does, though, with its cruel impositions – its impact on mobility, energy levels and constant biting with pain – is it makes everything in life harder than it ought to be, which is also what depression and anxiety do to anyone.

These conditions do feed into one another. Over time, it's no surprise to find yourself worn down, worn out, dealing with heavy thoughts and emotions, feeling alone and lonely, defeated by trying to open a screwtop bottle or make the bed.

It's vital you speak to your doctor if you're struggling to cope mentally. Some people think they shouldn't 'bother' the doctor unless it gets to a point where they begin to have suicidal thoughts - but please, don't wait for those to come along. They might not. You can be crippled by depression and not want to kill yourself. I know. But, if you are depressed, of course you are at greater risk of what the medical profession calls 'suicidal ideation' – which is, getting to a point where you start giving space in your head to thoughts of suicide. Anxiety and depression are treatable in more effective ways than fibro currently is, though. It might be that the FMS led to you getting depressed, which means it isn't a symptom, it's a consequence that can be addressed. Don't decide for yourself what constitutes a worthy topic to bring up with your doctor. Let them know where you're at, then they can discuss with you how to make life easier to manage. This could involve antidepressants but it might not.

Antidepressants have a certain stigma attached to them, with people thinking you're on them for life from your first prescription or they have horrible side-effects. All drugs have potential side-effects, not all of them manifesting in every person (if they did, the drugs would be pulled from the market) but most of any unpleasantness – rashes, tummy aches, nausea and so on – will go away after a short period of acclimatisation. Your first prescribed antidepressant might prove unsuitable, in which case your doctor can prescribe another to try. Or another. There's no one size fits all. Back when I took antidepressants, I think I must have gone through four different ones before my doctor found one I could tolerate. I recall one of the antidepressants I tried gave me an alarming facial tick around one eye, reminding me of the fictional TV detective, Columbo. I stopped taking that one fairly quickly!

Whether you stay on antidepressants for a year, two years or ten, that's all decided in conversation with your doctor over time. It depends on how you're feeling and what's going on in your life. I was on antidepressants for a period of five years. In that time, they helped me deal with some major difficulties and enabled me to find my way out of the depression.

FMS was once seen as an inflammatory disorder, then the prevailing view morphed into it being a disease of the central nervous system. Now a view of it as a 'biopsychosocial' disorder is gaining traction in medical circles, and it seems to me doctors are on the right track with this new approach because, even though I'm a layman, it makes the most sense to me. That long word, biopsychosocial, means FMS involves complex interactions between factors that are social, psychological and biological. Your body influences how you engage with your environments, your environments (including work and social activities) impact on your body, your mind is operating under these stressors that are physical and social and this leads to mental health issues to contend with which themselves make the other aspects worse. It's like one big horrible feedback loop. Or a frenzied feeding session in the pirahna tank.

You might find yourself on antidepressants not because you're suffering from depression but resulting from having FMS. Or, you might find the medicine prescribed to treat your depression also has an effect of reducing the severity of your fibro symptoms. This is because many of the drugs found to ease fibro pain were originally developed to treat depression and anxiety. Research into FMS has found, in the simplest terms, that its home in the brain is the same area associated with those other two conditions.

Why do so many people associate mental health problems with some perceived fault of their own? It doesn't make sense and it isn't helpful. It goes back centuries, to the days when people with mental health issues were called crazy and locked up. Institutions, such as the infamous Bedlam, would charge admission fees for people to come and watch the inmates – for inmates they were – as if they were animals in zoos. People have been making other people with mental health problems feel bad for centuries. It's not your fault, you aren't broken and you shouldn't take crap from anyone – including yourself.

Times have changed for the better but there's still a long way to go. Look at some of the words in common usage, just in casual conversations: crazy, bonkers, mental, not right in the head, not quite the shilling, mad, tapped… Words matter, as do opinions and general attitudes. You're free to challenge the language others use or not, but regardless you need to care about and for yourself, and not be bothered by what other people say. This can take time but they aren't living your life. You are.

It's important, if you think your mental health is suffering, not to beat yourself up about it. Getting help can begin with talking to your closest friend over coffee. Broaching the subject of what's going on inside your head with a medical professional can be a daunting prospect, so in the first instance having an informal chat with someone you know well and trust can really help, in advance of the appointment you need to make to see your doctor. The first time you open your mouth and let the truth come out can be scary. You can invite your friend along to your doctor's appointment if you want, if you think their presence by your side will help you get your words out.

If it's you listening to someone else share their story of depression and anxiety, don't let your empathy carry you away. You can be supportive and offer sympathy and advice without going away from the conversation with a head full of worry. Taking on board someone else's problems is the last thing you need. It won't make you more effective as a helper. Also, don't ever tell someone what medication they should be on. You're not a doctor or, even if you are, you're not your friend's doctor. Leave medication decisions to the confidential chats that take place between patient and doctor. What works for one person won't work for another. Besides, nobody is asking or expecting you to be an amateur pharmacist. Just be there for the people who need you.

Make sure, when you do give advice, that you're actually being asked to do that. Some people just need someone to listen and understand. A friend of mine no longer references her chronic health conditions on social media because she says she isn't doing it to get advice but just to share her life with friends, only she ends up getting 'healthsplained' as we refer to it - well-meaning advice gets posted in the comments, offered up by people who don't pause to think and instead carefully outline what my friend ought to be doing to manage her health problems. At best it's annoying; at worst, it's insulting. My friend no longer feels able to write posts about a huge part of her life. As she says, "If I want advice, I will say: I'd like some advice."

Feelings of depression and anxiety are always going to be worsened by the experience of chronic pain at the same time, but there may be other circumstantial factors in your life making things worse for you. You could be dealing with relationship problems or stressing about exams and money, or a host of other things life throws our way. When those issues and worries are dealt with, it doesn't always follow that the psychological upset disappears overnight. Think about the ripples in a pond when you throw a stone, how the ripples continue long after the stone has sunk to the bottom. When we suffer bereavement, the grief doesn't evaporate as soon as the funeral is over. It can go on for a long time. Reaching out for support is a win-win-win-win scenario. I could put a few more wins in there, but you get my point. And it's never too late, so if you're seeking help at the end of a relationship great - but if your relationship ended ten years ago and you know you need help to get over it, then go get that help. No counsellor on Earth is going to tell you you've gone past a sell-by date.

There are lots of things you can do to help yourself, and they all get mentioned throughout this book, though none of them should be seen as substitutes for talking to a medical professional. It's important to address the problems you encounter when trying to get asleep and stay asleep; exercise when you can, little and often being better than trying to bust a nut on epic marathons; don't eat junk and keep yourself hydrated; and, consider getting into meditation and attending physical and talking therapy sessions.

A review of clinical trials involving over 3,500 people found just thirty minutes of mindfulness meditation every day provided some relief from stress, anxiety and depression. You'll find local colleges and community centres often run short courses in mindfulness practice, and they don't cost a lot considering the benefits you'll gain. I attended one, which ran for ten weeks. It was several years ago, and I gained a valuable daily practice that helps me deal with my pain and focus on what's important.

What is mindfulness? Well, in the simplest terms, it involves learning to be present in the moment, rather than distracted and 'running on autopilot'. You accept the thoughts and feelings in your mind, cultivating a non-judgemental attitude towards others and your own self. A lot of people think meditation involves emptying your mind, something they know they can't do or have tried to do, only to end up frustrated. It doesn't.

When you practice mindfulness, the last thing you should be trying to do is banish thoughts. You let them come into your head, acknowledge their existence and send them floating away again.

Sure, they'll come back, many of them, and that's okay. There's this idea prevalent in society that meditation means parking on your bum and doing nothing at all, but meditation is about training your mind to become more aware, not less. It won't turn you into an empty-headed zombie. The longer you practice mindfulness, the better your chances of seeing improvement in your symptoms. Nobody seems entirely sure why it helps, although a placebo (purely psychological) effect has been ruled out.

I've met people who would like a single magic pill to make all the bad stuff go away, just as long as they remember to take it once a day. The truth is, only a few of us might say it out loud but all of us want it. Unfortunately, that's never going to happen with a condition like FMS. It's a chaotic, variable disorder that requires you to fight it on several fronts. We talk of fibro like it's a single entity but it isn't. It's highly unlikely it has a single cause. All the different symptoms, physical and psychological, feed into each other. There's an undeniable connection between pain levels and where you're at in terms of your mental health. Depression and anxiety don't just go away on their own. Get help. When you do and it starts to work, not only will the dark shadow over your life start to lift but you should also find your fibro symptoms become at least a little less impactful than they were. Always take a little improvement in preference to business as usual.

I'm not tired, I'm exhausted

When I was younger, which I like to think wasn't that long ago, I could happily party all night. I had the energy, drive and enthusiasm for clubbing. I loved music, still do, but these days the tunes tend to be listened to at home and in the car. I might dance a little when I'm cooking in the kitchen but it's a rare thing to find me on a dance floor. There are conventions, weddings and big birthday celebrations where I will always try to strut my stuff, though, pain levels permitting. When I do dance, it's in the full knowledge I'll pay for it the next day, possibly the day after that and the subsequent one as well. I go well into energy overdraft just for having the audacity to try to have a good time.

Fibromyalgia is a mean party-pooper. As anyone who suffers from it will tell you, it does its very best to stop you socialising and having a life.

It's like the mean old man who comes out from his house and shouts at you when you're a kid for playing football on the street. You don't want any trouble, you're not doing anything wrong, he just wants to have a go. That's FMS – always looking to pick a fight with you. Imagine that old man coming out every ten minutes to shout at you, how that would wear you down. Fibro does much the same thing. It saps you of energy and when it isn't doing that, it's making your energy levels go up, down and all over the place. You make plans and cancel them at the last minute. You wake up in the morning with a list of things you want to do, only to find exhaustion hits after only one or two items have been completed, the rest of your day spent on the sofa feeling like a wilted flower.

FMS is a catch-all umbrella term for a specific collection of symptoms, each of which is associated with other illnesses as well. When you talk to fibro sufferers, they'll sometimes reference their fatigue as Chronic Fatigue Syndrome (CFS) but they're not usually correct. They will have chronic fatigue as a symptom, not CFS unless they've been diagnosed with that as well as FMS. CFS is a standalone condition also known as Myalgic Encephalomyelitis (ME). For all that FMS plagues us with a number of debilitating symptoms, it doesn't involve CFS/ME. Still, the chronic fatigue we experience is much the same as that endured by people who have had a diagnosis of CFS/ME. FMS and CFS/ME do, however, have significant differences.

CFS/ME is thought to manifest following influenza or other viral infections but it's not known for sure. Fibro, on the other hand, often begins to affect people after they've suffered injury or emotional trauma. There are specific sites of tenderness and pain in people with FMS, whereas people with CFS/ME don't have them. CFS/ME is often accompanied by swollen glands, fevers and other inflammatory problems but blood tests on fibro patients don't reveal inflammatory markers, or if they do it's because they have other health problems going on. CFS/ME has no link to Irritable Bowel Syndrome, whereas IBS is strongly associated with FMS. When it comes to sleep, FMS and CFS/ME both involve difficulty and disruption but research in Japan has found differences in what's going on 'under the bonnet'. People with CFS/ME experiencing muscular aches and pains can take non-steroidal anti-inflammatory drugs (NSAIDs) like aspirin and ibuprofen, and get some relief by doing so. NSAIDs have no pain-relieving effect for people with fibro.

If I've got sufficient energy when experiencing pain, I can still get from A to B and accomplish some (by no means all) tasks, just as long as I take something for the pain, grit my teeth and accept it's going to take me some time. If, on the other hand, I've got no energy at all because a bad episode of chronic fatigue is happening and I'm in pain, with the best will in the world I can't get anything done. There have been times when the chronic fatigue aspect of fibro has swung a wrecking ball through my social calendar. I don't get out socially anywhere near as much as I would like, thanks to this illness, but I can have one event I'm looking forward to in the next three or four months, prepare for it and maybe buy some new clothes, get excited as the date of the event approaches, and then, on the big day itself – wham! I'm out. I'm on the sofa. I can barely move. It's like I've left planet Earth and gone to another one entirely, where the gravity is much denser and weighs me down. Then come the text messages I have to send and phone calls I have to make, telling the truth even though it sounds like an excuse to my ears. I'm ill. Sorry, I won't be able to make it. I'm crushed. I'm disappointed and I've disappointed my friends. I feel all the more wretched. And then I make a conscious decision to stop feeling bad about cancelling, because it's not my fault I'm ill.

The chronic fatigue aspect of FMS forces you to become the most reluctant hermit. Everyone likes to spend some time on their own but on their terms, when making a choice. I hate the way chronic fatigue rules over me. What I don't allow it to do is impact upon how I see myself. I did, back at the start of this journey with fibro, but not anymore. Now, if negative thoughts about myself surface, I dismiss them for the nonsense they are.

People too often associate chronic fatigue, when fibro sufferers talk about it, with tiredness. There's really no comparison. You get tired for a reason. If you've been on your feet all day, working hard, dealing with the horrors of the daily commute, the way you feel when you get home, take off your coat and slump on the sofa - that's tiredness. If you've spent two hours of the weekend at the gym, using all the machines, working up a sweat, then you've gone shopping and maybe followed that with a dinner party for friends, by the time you hit the sack you're going to be tired. Whatever you've been doing with your day, a good night's sleep sorts you out and you wake up the next day without feeling tired. Chronic fatigue is completely different. Tiredness is an effect resulting from a cause or multiple causes; chronic fatigue is the effect resulting from no discernible cause. The person suffering from chronic fatigue doesn't need to have been doing anything at all to feel it. Or maybe they did a little and it proved too much. The feeling is much more intense and debilitating than tiredness.

Chronic fatigue involves not only exhaustion but also sleepiness (which does not equate to actually being able to sleep); muscle weakness; impaired reflexes and slowed responses to stimuli; difficulty making decisions and judging situations; mood instability; headaches and dizziness. It can also involve poor coordination; increased susceptibility to colds, flu and other infections; and, reduced motivation to do even the most basic things like getting out of bed and going to the shops. Some people report their chronic fatigue is accompanied by decreased appetite, while others experience cravings for foods they perceive, sometimes subconsciously, as being high-energy. However it manifests in the individual, we are comprehensively four-letter-worded by it.

Chronic fatigue can be a symptom of treatable disorders - thyroid problems, anaemia, to name but two - and, when they are successfully treated, the chronic fatigue goes away. There's no cure for it when part of FMS or CFS/ME. When you're exhausted, all you can do is rest until you feel energy returning to your mind and body. Sometimes a 'duvet day' will effect a turnaround but it can take several days, a week or even a month or more before the malaise lifts from you.

The detrimental effects of being sedentary (doing nothing) are well-known but while there's an easy remedy for those who are not ill but simply lazy – get off your backside, do some work, go for a walk – someone living with chronic fatigue can't have some sort of epiphany and just start doing. We can't magic up the energy. There's no possibility of a hallelujah moment, where you leap from your bed and make a firm commitment to running two or three miles every day from now on. You just can't do that. Chronic fatigue can't be addressed by developing a desire to do things. We already have that desire. We're incapable of acting on it because our bodies won't let us.

When we're as capable of being active as we can be, we end up compensating for the time we've spent doing very little, by doing too much. That puts us back at square one. We enter into energy overdraft, then find chronic fatigue returns to flatten us like trees in a hurricane. It's important, but much easier said than done, to pace ourselves on better days and in so doing hopefully keep the chronic fatigue at bay. It's not only hard to exercise control and restraint over how we use our energy but it doesn't always work and it often isn't possible to even try.

You do, over time living with FMS, gain understanding of how the disease and its symptoms such as chronic fatigue can be triggered. You adapt and learn to avoid actions and situations. You get a sense of what costs are attached to everything you do. Sometimes, though, life throws things at us that we have to deal with, knowing full well what will happen afterwards. There are crises to deal with, like family emergencies, the death of loved ones or a child being rushed to hospital with an injury. We can't possibly eke out our energies when bad and difficult things happen.

When my father died, I really don't know how I kept going and did what I did. I built up the biggest energy overdraft ever. My inner banker obviously proved generous in a time of tragedy, but eventually the debt had to be settled. The payback involved was severe, its intensity and duration commensurate to the length of time I'd kept going in necessary defiance of my illness. Were I to approach my inner banker for extra funds to make the bed, do the washing up or have a night out with friends, there'd be no hope of receiving the same generosity as I would with a 'big news' event. I suspect all that time I spent shuttling my mother to and from the hospital, sitting for hours by my father's bed, experiencing grief, organising the funeral, I was producing a special soup of hormones and other chemicals in my body, to keep me going. You just can't conjure up the same mix in everyday life or, for that matter, on demand in a conscious way.

"You look tired," people will say. I don't know why. Did anyone, in the history of the world, ever feel better for someone pointing that out? Sure, when the chronic fatigue is getting me down - sorry, no, not getting me down, flooring me - I'm going to look tired to you. But I'm not tired, I'm exhausted. Even thinking can be too much. I love to read but there's little chance of that when chronic fatigue has me floating away, halfway through a paragraph. You might think me antisocial, or that I can't be bothered with you, when I won't answer the phone. It isn't a case of won't. I can't. The phone would feel heavy in my hand, and I wouldn't be able to concentrate on what you had to say to me. On days disrupted by chronic fatigue, other people to me can sound like the adults in the Peanuts cartoons, muffled and indistinct. I'd rather hide away than risk appearing rude because how I represent myself in the world matters to me. Chronic fatigue consumes everything. All you can do, which isn't what you want to do, is go to bed and sleep. It isn't any better than the usual FMS sleep, either.

Eating healthy food, making sure you drink lots of water, not pushing yourself hard… These things make sense for everyone. They won't stop you having chronic fatigue episodes. Eating junk, being dehydrated and dashing about the place will provoke your symptoms, sometimes not the next day but the day after. The best advice on dealing with chronic fatigue doesn't involve medications, diet, exercise or anything you can physically do. It relates instead to how you see yourself. Acceptance is how you deal.

This illness isn't your fault.

You aren't lazy.

You're not useless.

I've had some humdinger negative statements about myself enter my head from time to time. I've learned to banish them, and focus on positives even when I'm feeling like a bag of crap slammed against a brick wall. My positives won't all be the same as yours. I remind myself of the kindness I show to other people and animals, that I have an imagination and am creative, that I have good friends and was blessed to be raised by loving parents. These are things I can take pride in, and draw strength from on the weakest of days. You might have brought wonderful children into the world or be a fantastic, loyal friend.

The great things about us shouldn't be diminished by chronic fatigue taking us out of circulation from time to time. We mustn't let it rob us of our self-respect and self-esteem. If we didn't have enough of those to begin with, there's no better time than right now to start cultivating a kinder, gentler, more generous approach to our own selves.

How amazing is it that we get knocked down and get back up again? There's strength involved in that, not weakness. If you need to do nothing because chronic fatigue demands it, then do nothing. It will pass, eventually. Brighter, more capable days ahead are guaranteed. Their value and usefulness to you isn't in any way lessened by the fact that more chronic fatigue episodes will come along later. I've developed a deep appreciation of the 'can-do' days. People who enjoy wellness as a constant, I doubt they're as keenly aware of the blessing of good health as someone for whom feeling well is an occasional, even fleeting phenomenon. On good days I can smile just because I'm alive and not feeling fatigued or in pain.

If you find your mental health is suffering because of chronic fatigue or any other symptom of FMS, talk to someone, please. Be it a friend or therapist in the first instance, it helps.

Are you what you eat?

From when I was a kid all the way through to my mid-thirties, I could eat anything at all and stayed skinny. I wasn't always eating things that were good for me, especially when walking home from school having popped into the sweet shop to spend my pocket money. It was just that fat and sugar didn't collect around my waist because I was active and had a fast metabolism. At the age of 23 I became a vegetarian and remain so to this day. It meant I had to start thinking more about food, what went into it, to make sure I didn't inadvertently eat anything containing meat or fish. As well as meat and fish, a lot of sweets went off the menu because they contained porcine (pig) or bovine (cow) gelatine or a red colouring produced by boiling female cochineal beetles.

When you're a vegetarian or vegan (the latter descriptive meaning eggs, honey and dairy are also off the menu), people tend to assume you must be eating healthily. It isn't necessarily true because a lot of V-labelled food is now available to buy that is convenient, fast and doesn't contain any animal product but is as unhealthy and ultra-processed as a lot of the stuff available to omnivores. Whether you're vegetarian, vegan or an omnivore, the choice before you is the same: to eat food made from fresh ingredients or high-fat, high-salt, high-additive junk. Most of us try to consume the more virtuous choices but inevitably, from time to time, we go for the quick and easy.

When young, what you eat isn't likely to show any damage on the outside but you've no idea what's being done to the inside of your body until problems surface later in life. The only exception, being both visible and fairly quick to manifest, is weight gain. Obesity has become a problem even for very young children and teenagers. Only now are we starting to see governments, slowly and reluctantly because they don't want to upset big business, demanding manufacturers cut sugar and fat levels in what they produce. But when it comes to other diseases, it can be after decades of thoughtless eating that the consequences are realised.

Around the age of 35 I began to put on weight as my metabolism began to slow, which it inevitably does as we get older, although exercise temporarily speeds it up. I didn't put on a lot of weight but it was enough to take me out of the 'skinny' category and my days of being able to eat without apparent consequence were over. I was happy to go up a jeans size because I'd spent years, ever since my early teens, wishing I could gain some weight. Later, when my jeans started to feel a bit tight around the waist again, I realised I had to act or I would just keep getting bigger. I had to start paying attention to what foods I ate, and how much I ate. This coincided with an increased awareness of just how much rubbish goes into a lot of food we buy from supermarkets. Again, whether you're omnivorous, vegetarian or vegan, we're all equally likely to come across chemical preservatives and flavourings, artificial sweeteners and excessive amounts of salt and sugar unless everything we eat is hunted in the woods or dug up from clean unpolluted soil. Weight concerns aside, I wanted to eat – and grow – more healthy food, preferably organic as and when I could afford to do so.

By the time I got my diagnosis of fibromyalgia, I was eating healthily most of the time. My weakness was crisps (Americans call them chips and what we in Britain call chips, they call fries). I ended up refusing to buy multipacks and only buying occasional single packs. When I did buy multipacks I'd been able to wolf the lot in just a day or two. Not good. Other than crisps, I ate a lot of vegetables and fruits, way above the number of daily portions recommended by the government. I think I excused the crisps because I was doing so well with the fruit and veg, which was of course a ridiculous approach but not one I think is that unusual. I didn't have a lot of money at the time, so organic purchases were rare but I made an effort to buy locally produced foods as much as possible. I started to notice that some foods, though, no matter how healthy they were supposed to be, didn't seem to agree with me at all.

Bread, be it brown or white, artisan or mass-produced, was guaranteed to make me swell up like a balloon. If you can tolerate bread, it's better if it's properly made with traditional ingredients and using traditional methods - unlike the ultra-processed stuff that is pre-sliced, wrapped in plastic and by far the most popular kind bought today.

Since the 1950s, wheat has largely been harvested before it has a chance to ripen, so that it contains more gluten. Gluten is a mix of two proteins. It makes bread rise and more of it in the flour means bread will rise faster, which means mass production is speeded up. Modern cheap bread is pumped full of air, fat, sugar and salt as well as preservatives and various other chemicals, thanks to the work of scientists at the British Baking Industries Research Association in the early 1960s. It isn't just white bread but also wholemeal and 'brown' breads the production of which has been accelerated. As well as using wheat containing more gluten, the 20th Century manufacturing process - so different to traditional methods - also involves adding extra gluten to strengthen the flour.

One theory put forward for an increase in gluten intolerance and inflammatory diseases is that this radical agricultural shift that took place is the cause, introducing a lot more gluten to the diet. Gluten is in a heck of a lot of food. If you're sensitive to it you can forget anything containing wheat or coated in breadcrumbs. Less obviously, gluten is used in foods you don't associate with bread at all. For anyone with gluten intolerance or Coeliac Disease (which involves a dangerous hypersensitivity to gluten), paying attention to the ingredients on labels is always necessary.

My parents were old school when it came to bread. Born into families that didn't have a lot of money and living through the days of rationing, they would always tell me that, 'bread fills you up'. Yes it does, which means it stops you feeling hungry when there's nothing else to eat. The bread they grew up with, however, wasn't like that consumed by so many people in quantity today. Modern bread made with early-harvested wheat, no matter what the manufacturers claim, is as healthy an eating proposition as sawdust. Yet my father could never understand why my meals weren't accompanied by a couple of slices of bread, once I'd made the decision to cut it out altogether. Bread is deeply entrenched in many people's lives as a staple food. It isn't anywhere near as popular as it once was, though.

I don't want to entirely demonise bread. It can be made with other grains like spelt and buckwheat. Spelt does contain gluten but can be tolerated by people with mild gluten issues better than regular, post-1950 wheat. Buckwheat doesn't contain gluten. Bread marketed as gluten-free is available, made using buckwheat and other alternative flours (rice and coconut flour are often used). You do need to be watchful when it comes to how many gluten-free prepared food products you consume, as they can contain more sugar and fats than the foods they are substitutes for.

I've no axe to grind or banner to wave when it comes to people eating meat and fish. We all have the right to make our own choices and I've no interest in judging anyone for any reason. My own long-standing vegetarianism has moved closer to veganism as time has gone by. I'm an 'almost-vegan' because the pain and other symptoms of my FMS have proven to diminish in severity and frequency by cutting out dairy, which for me was the only significant animal-derived food group left after meat and fish were rejected. I consumed dairy – milk and cheese – for years after my last fish and meat meals. It hasn't been easy giving up dairy as well. It hasn't been the total nightmare I thought it might be, either.

One of the reasons dairy should be avoided or at least significantly reduced if you have chronic pain is sugar-related, because lactose, which may cause inflammation, is a type of sugar. Dairy produce also aggravates Irritable Bowel Syndrome and can cause bloating and digestive difficulties because of a protein in milk called casein, which some people find hard to process. Thankfully, non-dairy milks such as soya, almond, coconut and rice are much more easily sourced today from supermarkets than they were just a few years ago. It takes time to get used to them, and you might find some types and brands, when added to coffee in particular, don't result in something that looks appealing. I've yet to find a soya milk that doesn't turn my coffee into a curdled unappealing mess but almond and coconut milks don't cause any problem with how my coffee looks. None of these alternative milks contain anywhere near as much fat as cow milk, so coffee and tea can appear darker than you're used to.

The only reason I'm not 100 per cent vegan is because I sometimes eat eggs. They're always free-range and cruelty-free because they're from the rescue hens I keep as pets.

Eggs are an excellent source of protein and many vitamins and minerals, and are not thought to impact on FMS symptoms. Meat and fish are not considered problem foods when it comes to FMS, either, at least not unless they're in junk food. If you prepare, cook and eat meat and fish, carry on if that's what you want to do. If I were to insert a personal request here, it would be to source your meat from local producers, aiming for organic and avoiding meat from animals that have been factory-farmed. Choose meat from animals that got to live as nature intended. And don't forget, fish are often factory-farmed in confined spaces as well as animals such as chickens.

The number one food and additive we're told we should avoid when we have chronic pain is sugar. I hold my hands up: I don't consume a lot of sugar but the prospect of trying to cut it out entirely – and forever - fills me with horror. I know many people have done it successfully but I can't imagine a life without any added sugar at all, and I'm no sweet tooth. But you can curb your intake rather than go for total abstinence, and generally be a bit cleverer about how you get your sweet hits.

I've reduced my sugar intake in a number of ways. I cut out chocolate in all its many guises (it's dairy, after all). Whenever I find myself missing it, I remind myself that sugar increases inflammation, accelerates ageing and ramps up hypersensitivity to pain. I don't add sugar to tea or coffee. I don't eat biscuits. I don't generally consume fizzy drinks such as colas and lemonade (not only is the sugar bad but carbonated drinks are thought to exacerbate our digestive and bowel symptoms). I don't eat candy.

There's bound to be sugar hidden away in some of the foods I occasionally consume but I'm taking in considerably less sugar in my daily diet than the average Joe. While that's the way it has to be because I've got FMS, I do find it difficult and suspect I always will.

Chemicals with long, often unpronounceable, names are in so many food items these days. Checking the ingredients on tins, packets and bottles can be eye-opening. Artificial additives, preservatives and sweeteners are either completely benign or highly toxic, depending on who you speak to. Aspartame is the one that gets the worst press. I'm glad to have discovered long ago I've a sensitivity to it that makes avoiding it necessary.

Chemical additives are used to colour food, make it taste 'better' and last longer than it would if nature had its way. They're found not only in foods you might easily identify as ultra-processed, but also many preserved and cured meats or applied to salads. Nitrates and nitrites are common preservatives known to cause headaches, inflammation and fatigue. Dyes used in food can induce nausea, fatigue, headaches and vomiting. Monosodium glutamate (MSG) is a flavour booster added to many pre-packaged foods and takeaway meals. MSG has been shown to provoke our pain receptors and consuming it leads to an excess of glutamate in spinal fluid, which worsens fibro symptoms.

The best ways to avoid artificial additives, preservatives and sweeteners are:

(1) cook with fresh ingredients.

(2) eat raw organic food that hasn't been sprayed or injected.

(3) steer clear of sweets, processed meats and fast foods.

I never said it was easy. Nor attainable every single day in every circumstance.

When we have FMS, we're supposed to avoid fried food but, like sugar, I'd say lessening your intake is preferable to doing nothing at all and more likely achievable than complete abstinence. The problem with frying is it often involves trans fats, which are attractively dumped on our bellies and waists, and clog our arteries.

As a general rule, many of the foods you enjoy fried can be prepared in other ways such as boiling or cooking in the oven. It's a rare event when I take the frying pan out of the cupboard, being more likely to use a wok for stir-frying vegetables and even then only a couple of times each month. When using a wok I only need to use a fraction of the vegetable oil when compared to what goes into a frying pan. I avoid branded composite oils (where there's a mix of different oils in the bottle) and instead use coconut oil. With salads I'll generally use an extra-virgin olive oil, maybe with a splash of balsamic vinegar.

I'm not much of a drinker. I don't drink at home when I'm on my own and don't get out to clubs and pubs much because of my FMS and diverticular disease symptoms but, when I do, yes, I like to have a drink. And when I say 'a drink', I probably, in all honesty, and I must be honest in a book (it's a rule I follow), mean several. Enough to be just a little bit silly without getting to the point where I'd fall over and puke. Over the course of a year I drink far, far less than a unit a week.

Alcohol - any quantity, consumed at any time - is something you're supposed to avoid entirely when you suffer from chronic pain. It contains a heck of a lot of sugar, for one thing, and its dehydrating effect can trigger cramping, increasing the severity of IBS symptoms.

But hey. FMS robs us of anything and everything it can get its grubby, pain-inducing hands on. Allow us the occasional defiant act of enjoying ourselves, eh? Whether that's drinking with friends or going for a long walk, we FMS sufferers know that everything has a price on it.

When I've had even just a couple of drinks, I've downed them in the knowledge that, for a few days after, I'll experience worsened chronic fatigue and bowel pain. I don't get hangovers, drinking a couple of glasses of water before I go to bed whether I've been drinking alcohol or not, but then I don't drink enough during a night-out to risk a hangover anyway.

If you're going to have a gin and tonic or pint of ale every now and then, or even several, don't let anyone try to put you down for doing so. There exist in society people who think they are trying to do good by others who live with disabilities and illnesses by telling them what they should and shouldn't be doing. Is this wise? Are you sure you want to be doing this? Have you considered… Really, it's an ego boost for them and much, much less impactful on their own lives than going the whole Mother Theresa, packing their lives into one suitcase and moving to a poor country to pat starving children on the head while saying 'there, there'. Don't allow yourself to become someone else's pet project in any situation, especially when it comes to the decisions that are yours and yours alone to make. The most objectionable thing anyone can do to someone with a disability or chronic illness is try to take away their right to independent thought and decision-making, or challenge everything they say or do on the basis that their perceived weaker state means they cannot be trusted to run their own lives with diligence and self-care.

It's much harder for you when the overwhelming and suffocating concern comes from parents and other loved ones. My own mother doesn't like me doing pretty much anything that involves me going away and enjoying myself. She worries and I can't stop her doing it, but I do find myself having to offer reassurances much of the time and, occasionally, firm dismissals. She's got it into her head that I'm like thin, easily shattered glass because of my FMS. I've never given her or anyone else that impression. Everyone who knows me understands me to be tough and durable – my mum too, underneath her worries. Be patient with people whose love and care for you is genuine; communicate clearly but firmly, with kindness. You love them too, after all.

Okay, so we've covered all the wonderful yummy food and drink you can't or shouldn't have. Sorry about that. Are there any foods especially good for us when we suffer from chronic pain? The answer to that is yes. Avocados are a bit of a health craze at the time I'm writing this. They're not only tasty and diverse in their uses but they're packed with healthy fats and pain-relieving vitamin K. I use them in fruit and vegetable smoothies, in salads and on my gluten-free, wheat-free toast. I know, that statement makes me sound like such a hipster ready to post pictures of my food to Instagram but really, those who do that sort of thing have hijacked healthy eating and made a joke of it to others. Just because something is trendy doesn't mean it isn't good.

Dark leafy greens such as kale and spinach work to reduce something called 'oxidative cell stress' in the body, which damages cells, proteins and our DNA. Oxidative cell stress has been associated with a number of illnesses including FMS, diabetes, Alzheimer's disease, insomnia, anxiety and cancer. It can accelerate ageing too.

Like, wow. Get eating that kale. Hipster stereotypes be damned. Kale can be consumed in many ways, my preference being to use it in stir-fries and smoothies. Some people find kale to be a little on the bitter side or too tough for their liking, even when cooked. In comparison, spinach is a gentler, even sweeter flavour. I love spinach because it's incredibly versatile and very good for you. I eat it raw and cooked, in smoothies, stir-fries, casseroles and soups.

Wild salmon is a particularly good source for omega-3 fatty acids, which fight inflammation. Vegetarians and vegans are too often told that they're probably going to be deficient in omega-3 but it's no more likely the case than it is among the omnivorous population. Vegan-friendly (and therefore vegetarian-friendly) omega-3 capsules are available. The omega-3 is extracted from cultivated algae. It's also found in flax, chia and hemp seeds, as well as seaweed, mustard oil, beans, berries, honeydew melon, mangoes, wild rice and various herbs and spices.

Cherries are anti-inflammatory, containing lots of antioxidants, but I don't mean the sugar-coated ones you'll find on top of a Bakewell tart. Lemons and ginger are also said to be anti-inflammatory, along with the spice turmeric. Last, but definitely not least among the foods recommended if you suffer from chronic pain, come whole grains. These contain complex carbohydrates the body converts to energy slowly, which might help smooth out the peaks and troughs of chronic fatigue symptoms. Most grains are gluten-free, though not the most commonly eaten. If you need to avoid gluten, steer clear of barley, rye, wheat and most oats unless they come clearly labelled as gluten-free (oats often being contaminated with wheat).

I didn't change my diet overnight, other than when I became a vegetarian. With everything else – cutting down sugar, ditching dairy, eating new foods – I took my time, focusing on one before moving forward, having achieved my aim, to tackle another. If you're someone who responds well to making drastic overnight changes, then go for it when it comes to cutting out foods perceived to be harmful and introducing those said to be beneficial for fibro sufferers. If that's you, then great. I just don't think there are many people who would quickly, easily and comfortably embrace a whole new way of approaching their food and drink.

Out of everything, two changes stand out to me as being worthy of having priority status. Those are cutting down on sugar and ditching junk food. If you're going to start anywhere, start with ticking these off your list - and I do recommend you take action on the food and drink front. Not only is there the prospect of your FMS symptoms being eased somewhat, but you'll be improving the general health of your organs as well.

Do make sure you enjoy your food. It's best not to focus on all the things you should avoid and instead approach what you can eat, established and new foods, with a positive attitude of curiosity. What is this? How do I prepare it? What recipes can I find in books and on the Internet? What's quick to make and what's going to take me a while? You might be surprised how creative and inventive you can be, once you embrace change. If you find it hard, though, tell yourself that's okay. Because it is. If you occasionally break the rules you set for yourself, that's okay too. There are times when I get fed up and have an immense craving for foods I know do me no favours. I eat them knowing exactly what they'll do to me the next day. At the time I'm eating them, I don't care. I'm enjoying them. The day after, it's a different story. This is just human nature manifesting. I'm not going to feel immense guilt over occasional lapses, just the pain that comes with them. And hey, look. They do kale crisps now!

It's my belief that the fresher, rawer and 'cleaner' the food you consume, the better your health will be: lots of fresh fruit and veg, salads, organic and ethical meat and fish, free-range eggs... The science is going to be on the side of the processed food industry as a rule but, in practice, many people with different ailments report improvements in their symptoms when they start to be more aware of what they eat and cut out the rubbish.

I occasionally get grief from militant omnivores who think my choices are somehow a judgement on them. They assume I'm claiming some kind of moral superiority when I'm not. What I eat is nobody else's business to judge me on, or criticise me for. I won't stand for it, so why would anyone else? I don't really care what you eat. It's not my business. My point is, you should think about what you eat and how it impacts upon you and the world around you. What decisions you make following on from those thoughts are entirely your own.

Support

I remember attending a support group meeting organised through the hospital where I received my fibromyalgia diagnosis. It was for people whose diagnosis was recent, and when I got there I was the only man in the room. There were around twenty-five women, the majority of them aged between 35 and 55. Because I'd done some research beforehand, I knew it was likely there wouldn't be many men there but being the only one still managed to surprise me. It wasn't that I had any problem at all with the other attendees based on gender or anything at all. We all had fibro, but our life experiences were going to be markedly different. My sense of being separate from everyone else there was only made worse by every speaker who entered the room being female as well.

The presence of even just one other man, no matter his age or background, would have signalled to me that I wasn't alone in being male and having fibro. How reassuring and affirmative it might have been to meet other guys 'in the same boat' as me! I've since met other guys with fibro, online and off. We do find, whatever our differences - social, political, cultural, sexual - we are able to help each other, often in small but meaningful ways.

I didn't get a lot out of my two hours at the hospital that day. It wasn't the fault of anyone there. I'd already done my research, so a lot of the things that were said weren't new to me. They were new to plenty of other people, of course. It was great for them. But at least I gave it a try. I turned up. A lot of men feel unable to reach out for help when they're suffering in any way - physically, mentally, socially, financially. God knows we need support. Depression impacts upon millions of men the world over. In the UK alone suicide is the biggest killer of men under the age of 45. Male loneliness, too, has become something of an epidemic. We need, as a society, to tackle the underlying reasons why men don't reach out for the support they need - and why there isn't enough help out there for us to find when we do look for it.

When my fibro symptoms first fully manifested, I was at the tail end of a relationship that, as I've referenced earlier in the book, had become utterly, irredeemably toxic. I don't think I'd ever felt so lonely before, so isolated. Yet my response to the physical and emotional pain was to isolate myself even more. In the first two years after becoming single again and living with fibro, I largely cocooned myself inside my house and rarely attempted anything social. I could go several days without even speaking to another human being. Most of the time I only spoke to my mother and father, and checkout staff at the supermarket. Writing about this now, looking back, I find the extent of my separation from the world, from other humans, astonishing.

I didn't become a hermit on purpose, at least not consciously so. If I hadn't had my pets to look after, elderly parents reliant on my visits and care, and an exceptional best friend, I've no doubt at all I'd have considered taking my life. What stopped me was being haunted by thoughts of who would fill my shoes where my parents were concerned, what would happen to my beloved animals with me gone, and what would my best friend do without me? Not once, during that terribly difficult time, did I ever think me being me was a reason not to end it all. I can remember not caring about myself at all. I held on for others, human and animal. Thank goodness I had those people and pets in my life, because they kept me here until I rediscovered the sense of my own life being as important as everyone else's.

For the longest time I had no ability to see myself as having a worthwhile existence, not weighed down as I was by emotional devastation with chronic fatigue and pain coursing through my body, making me feel like an old man whose life was over. I was just marking time, putting one foot in front of another, then again, just to get through each day.

While the fibro hasn't gone away, the mental and emotional difficulties are in the past. Things only changed for me when I decided they had to change, and reached out.

Change is pretty much the only constant in the universe. If you take your hands off the steering wheel when driving a car, the vehicle isn't going to continue on in a straight line. It's more likely to start veering off to the left or right, until it hits something. If you take charge, though, the direction of the vehicle is determined by you. This is absolutely true of our lives as well as cars. Had I not decided change directed by myself was necessary, eventually my mental health would have worsened, making suicide more and more likely. No matter how wretched you feel, you can always choose to take control and you must if you're going to stand any chance at all of getting through the dark tunnel to the light.

It takes immense courage to get out there when you're more inclined to hide away at home, and to speak to doctors and mental health professionals, but I believe the required courage resides in all of us. Reaching out for help involves acknowledging you're a vulnerable person, not only to yourself but to other people as well.

I'll say it now: I'm a vulnerable person.

I'm still a man.

I'm a man who will remain vulnerable for as long as FMS has no cure and no treatment that effectively masks all the pain and other symptoms associated with it. That vulnerability is both physical and emotional. I don't think a waking moment goes by when I'm not aware of it, from when I'm trying to open a tin or bottle and can't do it, through to those times when I want to try dating again but then baulk at the idea of having to 'come out' about my disability to someone I've only just met, because I don't want to invite judgement.

There was a time when the sense of my own vulnerability only served to weaken me further, depressing and demotivating me. Now, though, having acknowledged it, I own it fully and draw great strength and determination from the courage of my disclosure to myself and others. Vulnerability isn't a curse. It isn't a hole in the armour. Vulnerability is my superpower now I'm no longer scared by it, or ashamed of it. It used to scare the shit out of me, of course it did. I feel vulnerable writing this, knowing strangers the world over will read it. The vulnerability can't stop me, though. Not anymore. Dignity, self-respect, purpose and pride are waiting to be owned by you once you recognise your vulnerability is capable of showing you and others what strength resides within you. If a person has always had it easy, how are they ever to know what they're capable of?

Those of us living with FMS are often referred to as being 'fibro warriors' within the online FMS communities. I think that gloriously proud phrasing perfectly encapsulates how we should see ourselves: not as broken people unable to do this or that any more, not as victims afflicted by a terrible blight, but as courageous fighters instead, doing whatever is necessary to make something of our lives.

I'm a fibro warrior because I'm writing this book, for one thing. I write when I can. It's not easy but I do it. That's a fighter, not a loser. I'm a fibro warrior when I get out of bed every day, get washed and dressed, get out into the world and live my life. I'm a fibro warrior when I go to bed at night, eventually get to sleep only to be woken by pain, curse and wince, then do my best to sleep again. I'm a fibro warrior when I endure, when I triumph and even when I lose having given everything I could. I'm a fibro warrior because I chose therapy over endless misery. I'm a fibro warrior because I'm still here, years after my diagnosis, battling on.

It's so much better to see yourself as a warrior rather than a failure, useless and damaged. Those are horrible negatives. They keep you down. They aren't true. So much can be achieved in this world when we learn to be kinder to ourselves, prouder of ourselves, and choose to think more positively about who we are and what we manage to achieve in our daily lives. I'm not one for saying positivity solves every problem, cures every illness – it really doesn't – but negativity, turned upon our own selves, achieves nothing but harm. Please, banish that shit. If you give up, don't expect to win. I guarantee you won't get anywhere if you don't try.

Many of the issues men have, which prevent them from reaching out, originate in childhood. As little boys they're taught how men 'should' be, not only or necessarily in the home but also at school and socially. You're a sissy if you cry. You need to be strong. Boys have to be on top, in charge. Boys are doers. Get it done. Don't 'whinge'. These and other received messages are false and destructive. Women, too, back when they were young girls, were presented with lies dressed up as truth, from many different authorities in society, told how they should behave and even what they could or couldn't express interest in pursuing.

The key difference is, little girls aren't generally taught that emotional expression is unacceptable. Men are, though. We're all, to some degree, artificially constructed, with a layer of expectations deposited on top of our natural selves. We are conditioned. Throw away the rulebook because most of those rules were written when we still daubed things on cave walls. We owe it to ourselves to be honest in assessing who we are, what we are, where we've been. We need to bin those expectations received from others that don't serve us well at all.

When you were growing up, were you encouraged to ask for help? What happened when you did? The origins of a reluctance to ask for help - and the ability to ask for help easily - lie in our formative years. This applies to men and women. It's only by becoming fully aware of what went on in the past that we can begin to address what's going on in the here and now.

If you're at the point where you know you need help but don't know how to go about getting it, the first thing you might want to consider trying is a call to a disability helpline or the Samaritans. You don't have to be in crisis mode, or suicidal. These free services can offer you anonymity, advice and listening ears. You won't be judged and your problems won't be dismissed. Just one phone call, be it ten minutes long or an hour, can give you a huge psychological boost and the sense of having a plan for how to proceed in securing your recovery.

Therapy can be enormously useful in bringing down the barriers we put up. Those barriers are meant to be defensive but all too often prevent us from learning, growing and moving forward. A therapist offers a safe, supportive environment that is completely confidential. If you're dubious about it, commit to just six sessions and see how they go.

If you're okay with the idea of meeting people face-to-face, it's definitely worth looking into whether there are any FMS support groups meeting in your area. Making new friends who are also living with FMS, you'll find you don't need to explain your daily struggle. They just get it. The fact that they do can be incredibly refreshing, coming after years of trying to get others to understand. If walking into a room full of strangers is a scary prospect, check with the organiser beforehand whether it's okay to take along your best friend or partner to your first meeting. Alternatively, if you tell the organiser you're feeling a bit anxious, they'll probably be more than happy to greet you outside the room and have a chat before you go in.

The internet is an incredible resource for information and support, but should be approached with caution. Not everything you read on there is true – blog posts, news articles, comments and more can be filled with misinformation and even deliberate lies. A lot of material around FMS is written with an eye on drawing high visitor numbers in, with sensational headlines offering false hope rather than factual information. There are articles claiming you can lead a completely pain-free life if you eat this or that vegetable or fruit several times a day, every day. Others report 'cures' for FMS or theories as to its origins that have no basis in fact and no support from within the medical profession. I was incensed when I came across an article that claimed people with FMS suffered abuse in childhood. Some might. Many don't. I've already written, earlier in this book, that those who were abused as children in any way are more likely to develop FMS as adults but there's no certainty. You simply cannot say all people with FMS suffered abuse as kids. That isn't true. The post was shared far and wide, provoking many discussions and getting far more attention than it deserved. So we will have some people in the world who, when told you have FMS, will think you were abused as a child.

Still more pages online will blast this or that drug used in the treatment of FMS as damaging, when there's no scientific evidence behind the claim. It's easy for a stranger to tell you to stop taking your medication but incredibly stupid to do so unless under the instruction of your own doctor or hospital consultant.

You'll probably find well-meaning friends send you links to pages from time to time, asking, "Did you know about this?" or, "Have you tried this?" It always pays to keep in mind your friend is trying to be helpful and doesn't need a sarcastic or blunt comment flung their way, no matter how tempting it might be after being sent the same link seven times by seven different people.

Facebook, for all its many reported faults and concerns, remains a great place to find forums relevant to many topics, including FMS. When you're logged into it, using the search bar at the top to input 'fibromyalgia' will result in a list of pages and groups that might overwhelm you at first. Groups tend to be highly active, getting a lot of posts and comments every day. You ask to join them, or you're invited to do so, or a friend adds you to them (that last one really annoys me if I wasn't asked by the friend first). Pages are more static, involving comment discussions under posts made by a single person or team running the page. When it comes to pages, you click to 'like' them and the posts should then start to appear on your news feed. If they don't, return to the page and click on the 'follow' button sitting right next to the 'like' button.

I don't want to recommend specific groups or pages, although I belong to a number of useful Facebook groups filled with supportive, friendly people. I've also been a member of groups I've left within minutes of joining, having witnessed virtual brawls where people wrote abusive things aimed at each other and there appeared to be no admins willing to intervene and put a stop to bullying.

You can find FMS support groups and pages specific to your region and country as well as those welcoming new members from around the world. A good group has a well-thought-out list of rules you must read when joining, clearly outlining zero tolerance of bullying, racism and other nasty behaviours, informing you as to what is and isn't acceptable to post. It will have an admin or group of admins seen to operate fairly, without prejudice, and can be easily contacted in the event of any problems arising.

Don't expect admins to be available around the clock, though. They're always volunteers and never deserve anyone going full-on diva at them with a tantrum because a message wasn't replied to the same day it was sent. Patience and courtesy bring rewards, in that deploying them is far more likely to get you favourable responses. Rudeness and hostility will get you kicked out.

When it comes to medications, a responsibly-run group or page isn't going to permit members to recommend drugs to one another. It's one thing to talk about your own experience of being on amitriptyline or using CBD oil, but it's another thing entirely to advocate somebody else tries it. When it comes to cannabis, some groups prohibit discussion of it entirely because of its legal status varying from country to country. If they do, it will be stated in their rules.

You have to use the 'suck it and see' approach to find groups and pages that are a good, lasting fit for you. Read the About section on any group before you join, and remember you can leave at any time for any reason.

You might come across pages and groups that are, for want of better phrasing, 'anti-fibromyalgia', their purpose being to rubbish the experiences of those with fibro as being fake or wrongly diagnosed. They're easy to spot, so there's no risk of you joining them by accident. Don't let them upset you. It's a great big world and a great big internet, with lots of trolls (otherwise ordinary people who like to bully and upset others online) looking to wind you up. The very worst thing you can do is engage with trolls and argue with them. They love that. It's what they live for. Deny them their pleasure and focus on what's good and useful for you, which doesn't involve wasting time on idiots.

Twitter can be useful, though it's a very different experience to Facebook and can be challenging to get to grips with. Many FMS charities and campaign groups can be contacted directly on there, with lots of individuals living with fibro sharing useful and interesting links. Again, as with Facebook, you can encounter abusive trolls. Block them. Be respectful and courteous to others at all times, even if someone is trying to provoke you. Be mindful that, as with Facebook, you shouldn't assume articles shared on there are going to be factual. Fake news is the scourge of our times, after all.

I'm on Twitter - @ndrewHinkinson - and I'm there not only because I find it a useful resource for FMS but also it gives me the means to connect with like-minded individuals and organisations relating to my politics, interests and hobbies. You're very welcome to 'follow' me on there. You might not agree with every word I put out in my tweets but then, you won't agree with everything any individual says on Twitter, any more than you'd agree with every word your partner or friend has to say on any given subject. As with Facebook, patience and courtesy and respect are all essential. Sadly, not everyone displays those attributes and people are best avoided when they show themselves to be less than social on social media. I have an author page on Facebook (just search on there for my name) which I'd love for you to 'like' and 'follow' for news about my book projects and links shared to FMS articles you can trust as well as pertaining to my other interests, which range from books (obviously enough) through to keeping pet chickens (which I do, and wrote a book about).

When I did finally reach out for support, I was glad I did. I can't imagine anyone in need of help reaching out to phone counsellors, therapists, doctors and well-organised, reputable online forums and ever regretting doing so. I know I'm not alone in fighting this dreadful and mysterious disorder, this group of disruptive and life-changing symptoms. Despite the pain and difficulties, I have a good life and have learned a great deal from living with FMS. I've made some amazing friends who also live with this illness and whose life experiences, while very different to my own, have inspired me and continue to do so.

It was my hope, in writing this book, to explain and demystify FMS for those of us who live with it and for family and friends who want to understand and help us. In focusing on FMS through the prism of my own experience, I'll inevitably have left some things out. That's because I haven't experienced everything. I had no intention of listing every drug or covering every illness people might conceivably be dealing with alongside FMS. This was a book written by a patient, not a doctor. I don't write the prescriptions, I get them written for me. It's been about my own personal journey with FMS, what I've learned. If we only had books about medical conditions written by doctors, I don't think we'd gain understanding of what it's really like for people to live with disabilities, diseases and disorders.

Everyone's experience of FMS is going to be unique to them. We each have our own stories to tell and, regardless of whether you're a writer or something else entirely, we are all capable storytellers deserving of having people in our lives who will listen to what we have to say and work with us to make life easier for everyone. If you're living with FMS, as a fellow warrior fighting the fight, I salute you.

If you enjoyed reading this book, I'd really appreciate it if you could give me a few minutes of your time by leaving a review on Amazon and/or Goodreads (a social network for readers). It's not just so that I can afford to pay my rent, though of course I need to earn a living from my writing, but also because I want there to be better understanding in the world of what FMS is, how it affects people.

Keep hoping for a cure and know that research is ongoing. One day it will come. Be kind to yourself, and thank you for reading *my*fibromyalgia.

UK further info and help

Fibromyalgia Action UK National Helpline
0300 999 3333, Mon-Fri 10am-4pm
fmauk.org

UK Fibromyalgia
http://ukfibromyalgia.com

Arthritis Research UK - Fibromyalgia
0800 5200 520, Mon-Fri 9am-8pm
arthritisresearchuk.org/arthritis-
information/conditions/fibromyalgia.aspx

UK Disability Benefits Information
gov.uk/dwp

UK Disability Law Service
0207 791 9800
dls.org.uk

UK Citizens Advice - Disability discrimination
citizensadvice.org.uk/law-and-
courts/discrimination/protected-
characteristics/disability-discrimination

European Disability Forum
edf-feph.org

9 781982 995317